MASTER YOUR MIND

The More You Think

The Easier It Gets

By

D. E. Boyer

Disclaimer - Some names and identifying details have been changed to protect the privacy of individuals. I have tried to recreate events, locales and conversations from my memories of them. In order to maintain their anonymity in some instances I have changed the names of individuals and places, I may have changed some identifying characteristics and details such as physical properties, occupations and places of residence. Although the author and publisher have made every effort to ensure that the information in this book is correct, the author and publisher do not assume and hereby disclaim any liability to any party for any loss, damage, or disruption caused by errors or omissions, whether such errors or omissions result from negligence, accident, or any other cause.

Medical disclaimer - The author of this book is not a medical doctor or psychiatrist or psychologist. The author is not trained or certified in diagnosing or treating medical or psychiatric ailments of any kind, and the information in this book is not intended as a substitute for the medical or psychiatric advice of physicians and psychologists. This information in this book is not advice, and some authorities will have completely different opinions on how to manage their mental and physical health. Before taking any course of action mentioned in this book, the reader should consult with their health care provider for a thorough evaluation. Everyone is different and requires their own specific way of managing their mental and physical health, so the reader should regularly consult a physician or psychologist in matters relating to his/her health and particularly with respect to any symptoms that may require diagnosis, medical, or psychiatric attention. Every effort has been made to ensure that the information contained in this book is complete and accurate. This book is intended to provide helpful information for the general public. Please be

i

advised that the author and publisher are not engaged in rendering medical, health, psychological, or any other kind of personal professional services in this book. The information in this book should not be considered complete, and it should not be used in place of a call or visit to a professional or licensed therapist, medical, health, psychological, or other competent professional, who should be consulted before adopting any of the suggestions in this book. The information about vitamins, nutrients, drugs, and dietary supplements contained in this book is general in nature and does not cover all possible uses, actions, precautions, side effects, or interactions of any of these things described in this book, and a medical professional should be consulted before doing anything mentioned in this book. The information in this book is not intended to be medical or psychological advice for individual problems or for making an evaluation as to the risks and benefits of taking or not taking a particular drug, supplement, or other course of action. The author and publisher of this book disclaim all responsibility for any liability, loss or risk, personal or otherwise, which is incurred as a consequence, directly or indirectly, of reading or using this book in any way, and relying on any information in this book is solely at your own risk. In case of a medical emergency or if you are considering harming yourself, you should call 911.

For more information go to InfinitePotentialofYourMind@gmail.com

For my girls

Chapter 1

IT'S ALL IN YOUR HEAD

"Only that day dawns to which we are awake" -
Henry David Thoreau

The Bridge

Without purpose, our long journey through life will be meaningless, and peace and joy will escape us. But finding and maintaining purpose in our life is easier said than done. We can spend years believing that something matters, only to have its meaning suddenly slip away, leaving us wondering why it ever mattered in the first place. Then a few more years go by without purpose and we become numb to passion, forgetting what it feels like to really care about anything at all. Some people are born knowing their purpose, but many of us are unable to clearly see our path, or to be definitively drawn in the right direction. It will be difficult, if not impossible, to find our way while chaos is present in our mind. So we must develop the skill of managing this chaos if we are to have any hope of finding our true path. Once the chaos is controlled and our purpose becomes clear, then the harmony created by this process can open another dimension in our mind, a place where creative insights and magic moments transform our lives.

It's going to take some work, but those of us who prevail on our journey will ultimately find the road to peace and joy. Many of us will struggle along the way, and the things we do will often be twice as hard, and take twice as long as we thought, but the people who persevere will make it to their destination. There will also be a few lucky ones who slip through the cracks and automatically end up where they want to be, without ever having to endure the emotional slaughter of repetitive failures and starting all over again... again and again. If I've left anyone out, it's the ones who never make it at all. Some of these lost souls will take their own lives, and some will live long "lives of quiet desperation". In the end, the happiest people will be those who refuse to let their unfulfilled hopes and dreams turn into the whispered regrets that so many people utter with their last few breaths.

*

It's easy to remember how amazing my life felt when I was little, but by the time I turned forty-five years old, it was hard to forget how meaningless so many things in my life felt. As a child, the possibilities seemed endless, and ordinary things like the transformation of the seasons would always blow my mind. I used to love sitting on the porch on the first warm summer night of the year; listening to the sound of crickets and watching the light of the stars slipping through the treetops would send me into a reverie. But after four and a half decades of living, my sensory receptors and ability to experience awe had been beaten and battered, and I hardly noticed what day it was, let alone the season. If you had told me when I was little that when I grew up I would have one or two friends that I hardly talk to, a strained marriage, an unpleasant and unrewarding job, and no plans for the future, I would have said you were crazy. I would have said, "That's not me you're talking about; you must have me confused with someone else. When I grow up, my life will be just as amazing as it is now." I feel like I somehow let that child down because I really thought that I would be happier at this point in my life. I must have missed something important somewhere along the way, and if I could just start all over again, maybe I would be able to figure out where I went wrong.

I always knew there were many other people who, like myself, had trouble figuring things out. They never figured out how to stop making the same mistakes, over and over again. They never figured out how to

feel better, and how to think better. I knew there were a lot of people...
I just didn't know there were that many. That's why I was surprised at
what I learned when I was flipping through the paper one day. There
was a beautiful picture of the Golden Gate Bridge with the blue sky,
mountains, and ocean in the background. In front of it was a large
expanse of what appeared to be many different pairs of empty shoes,
hundreds if not thousands of them. I thought it was some silly work of
art, and there were people all around it taking pictures, but what it
turned out to be was a display of shoes representing all of the people
who killed themselves by jumping off the bridge during the 75 years of
the Golden Gate Bridge's history. There were 1,558 pairs of shoes in the
display. I understand that, every now and then, someone will want to
throw themselves off a bridge, but that seemed like a lot of people to
me. I also had no idea that there was a favorite spot, but the Golden
Gate Bridge is the most popular spot for committing suicide in the
country, and some sources state that it's the most popular site in the
world. It has some steep competition though, from the Nanjing Yangtze
River Bridge in China, which claims over 2000 suicides. Apparently,
jumping off a bridge is a popular choice for ending one's life, although
it wouldn't be my first choice.

The first person to jump off the Golden Gate Bridge did it about 3
months after it was finished being built in 1937. It was a 49-year-old
bargeman named H.B. Wobber who, right before he jumped, reportedly
told another man that he was walking with, "This is where I get off. I'm
going to jump." This man and all the others who jumped off the bridge
fell 220 feet over 4 seconds at a speed of around 75 miles per hour before
they hit the frigid water. I can't imagine how anything could be worse
than enduring this, but apparently many people think there is.

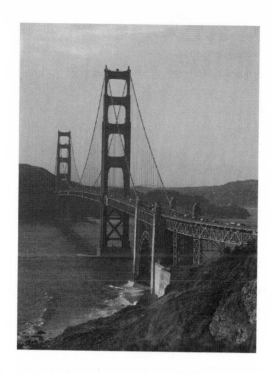

The official suicide count ended in 1995 because it was drawing too much attention from people who were considering suicide, and some of them were competing over which number jumper they were going to be. The total number of jumper deaths is now said to be greater than 1,600. August of 2013 was the worst month on record, when 10 people jumped off the bridge, 1 every 3 days. Not surprisingly, 2013 turned out to be the worst year ever for the bridge with 46 suicides. The year 1945 claimed the youngest person to jump off the bridge, 5-year-old Marilyn Demont, who was supposedly told to jump by her father, a 37-year-old elevator installation foreman who jumped right after her.

It's no surprise that if you do decide to jump, the odds are pretty good that you'll die. There have been a few lucky ones who survived and said they regretted jumping as soon as their feet left the bridge. Although one young woman, Sarah Rutledge Birnbaum, survived the first jump, but allegedly returned to jump again and died the second time.

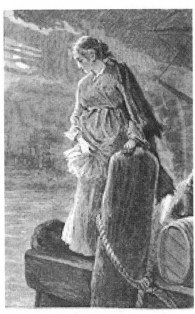

THE STREET GIRL'S END.

Most people don't realize how powerful their minds are, for better or for worse, and unfortunately, it's often for worse. The sad truth is that some people's minds are so dysfunctional that ending it all is the best solution they can come up with, and the statistics don't seem to be improving. Many people know of someone who has killed themselves or attempted to. According to the VA's latest Suicide Data Report, 22 veterans commit suicide every day. The latest student survey conducted by the Centers for Disease Control and Prevention revealed that 8% of teens said they had attempted suicide at least once in the previous 12 months. There's even a category for 10 to 14-year-olds; it's hard to imagine how someone who has only been alive for 10 years could even contemplate suicide, let alone successfully commit it. Overall, the total number of suicides has risen more than 30% in the last decade to an annual rate of 42,773, which averages out to about 117 people per day taking their own lives in this country alone. The largest increase in suicides was seen in adults aged 35 to 64, where suicide is the fourth most common cause of death after cancer, heart disease, and unintentional injuries such as car accidents. Males ages 45 to 64 are at the top of the list, holding the greatest percentage of all suicides.

This is a wakeup call for one of the largest portions of America's population. If you're a 50-year-old male, you now may have a better chance of putting a gun to your head and pulling the trigger than you do of dying in a car accident. Think about that the next time you're contemplating your life while driving to work in the morning. So instead of blowing your head off, you may as well take some time to figure out what's really going on in there, and learn what's been diminishing the return on your life. This will certainly require some soul-searching, and it may be a bit uncomfortable at times; but as Lewis Presnall said in his famous book, *Search For Serenity*, "No one can learn to be at home in his own heaven, until he learns to be at home in his own hell".

*

The power of our mind is greatly underestimated. Maybe underestimated isn't the right word though; "undervalued" might be a better word, judging from the cuts to mental health that have taken place over the years. According to the National Alliance on Mental Illness, 1 in 17 people in America lives with a serious mental illness such as schizophrenia, major depression, or bipolar disorder. Approximately 20% of youths ages 13 to 18 experience a severe mental disorder in a given year. The community services available for these people are disappearing at an alarming rate.

One would think that mental health would be more of a priority for the government, just looking at the increase in mass shootings that have occurred over the last decade. In fact, six of the twelve deadliest shootings in U.S. history have taken place in the last six years, and that doesn't even include the terrorist attacks. The gun control debate is complex and exhausting, but it doesn't take a rocket scientist to see that allowing anyone, let alone a terrorist, to purchase body armor and an A-K 47 should not be allowed. Yet congress can't pass the bill, and as the line between who's a terrorist and who isn't becomes more unclear, the bodies keep piling up, making mental health legislation even more of a priority. Whether you're born in this country or not, if you take joy in slaughtering large numbers of innocent men, women, and children, you're mentally disturbed and you shouldn't be able to buy a gun; but it's still pretty easy and that's a story for another book. Meanwhile, thousands of more people will die by their own hands due to the chaos in their minds. So as gun control continues to take center stage in congress and on the news, no one ever mentions the mental health side of the story and that perhaps maybe there's a connection. Sorry, I guess we find members of congress fighting over gun control far more exciting to watch on TV than hearing about people with mental illnesses getting help from the community, boring!! Mental illness is depressing, but don't take my gun away, I might need it to kill myself with it. Don't get me wrong, we bought a gun for protection because our neighbors were drug dealers and we thought they were going to kill us, but it's still hard to say if we're any safer with the gun in the house, or without it.

Couldn't we just spend a little more time trying to provide those 43,000 people who are going to kill themselves this year with mental tools that will help them realize that perhaps life is worth living? The answer always seems to be, "No, there's no money for that." The drug companies have found a way to profit from making people "feel better", so why can't congress realize that making people feel better will save this country billions of dollars in lost productivity alone? And do the drugs really make people feel better? Some studies show that the effects of antidepressants or anti-anxiety medication aren't any better than either a placebo or cognitive behavioral therapy. No one would argue that, if you're thinking about killing yourself, you should probably be on some kind of medication, and there are plenty of people out there that should be medicated and aren't. But I would also venture to say that there are a good number of people out there that are medicated and wouldn't need to be if they invested more time on their mind and body.

The third most frequently prescribed drugs are antidepressants. Some antidepressants have even been approved for adolescent depression; do you know any adolescents who aren't depressed? Jackpot!! Antidepressants are now pulling in over 12 billion dollars in sales; what on Earth did people do before them? According to the CDC, the rate of antidepressant use among people ages 12 and older increased by almost 400% over just a 15-year period; 11% of Americans ages 12 and older take antidepressant medication.

Here are a few other stand-out statistics from the Centers for Disease Control report on antidepressant use in this country:

*Overall, females are 2½ times as likely to take antidepressant medication as males.
*23% of women aged 40–59 take antidepressants, more than in any other age-sex group.
*14% of non-Hispanic white persons take antidepressant medications compared with 4% of non-Hispanic black and 3% of Mexican-American persons
*Less than 1/3 of persons taking a single antidepressant have seen a mental health professional in the past year.

Let's face it, we love popping pills and have for a long time now. It's quick; it's easy, and requires essentially no work on our part. Immediate gratification, what could be better than that? Speaking of immediate gratification, diazepam, otherwise known as valium, became quite popular when it was released in 1963 as an improved version of Librium (a drug which is used to treat alcohol withdrawal). That's what they put my mom on when she had her "nervous breakdown", and she was never the same again. Diazepam was the top-selling pharmaceutical in the United States from 1969 to 1982, with peak sales in 1978 of 2.3 billion tablets. Prescriptions of valium were down to only about 14 million last year; but have no fear, something else has taken its place. Valium's market rival Xanax has almost 50 million prescriptions, making it the most popular psych drug in America. That's almost 1 out of every 6 people taking anti-anxiety medication, and almost 1 in 4 women my age taking antidepressants. Everyone stop what you're doing and look around you; if you're not taking an antidepressant or anti-anxiety medication, someone sitting next to you probably is.

People should be required to do something other than simply taking an antidepressant, sitting back, and waiting for it to kick in. Pericles, one of the most famous generals in ancient Greece, once said, "With us it is no disgrace to be poor; the true disgrace is in doing nothing to avoid poverty." I would like to change this by replacing the word "poor" with the word "unhappy" and say that it's no disgrace to be unhappy; the true disgrace is in doing nothing to avoid unhappiness. Perhaps if we felt better, we wouldn't be so poor. So if we want to feel better, let's do something about it. It's unfortunate that we need to spend so much time making ourselves feel better; after all, there are so many other pressing matters at hand. But we do because if we don't start feeling better then we won't give a crap about anything else. We have to accept the fact that, in the words of Nietzsche, "Man is the only animal who has to be encouraged to live." So let's encourage ourselves, shall we?

First, we must take a closer look at what's really happening here. We could go on for years analyzing and debating the root causes of our unhappiness, but it doesn't take long to see what we all have in common in this area. Our inability to think well is at the top of the list of things we need help with, and no matter how many pills we take, none of them will help us with this. We have to fix this problem the old-fashioned way, by plowing through the layers of muck that have built up in our minds over the course of a lifetime.

No one ever taught us how to think; there are no classes in school that specifically teach us how to do this. It's just naturally taken for granted that thinking is automatic - that our minds are on autopilot and we will think the way we do now... forever. Fortunately, this is not the case. We now know that, if we put a little thought into it, we can control our thinking and vastly improve our lives in the process. But we have to teach ourselves how to discipline our minds, and this requires a clear understanding of how the mind works, as well as its relationship with the body. It also requires freeing the mind of chaos, because it's extremely difficult to control our thoughts when our minds are filled with chaos.

Some people are sick all the time, and they usually blame this on bad genes; but they can't blame it all on the genes. Perhaps the genes are getting their messages from the mind, and if there's chaos in the mind, there will be chaos in the body. The problem is that the majority of the things we say to ourselves are negative, and negative thoughts weaken our immune system, making us susceptible to disease. The number of thoughts each person has in a day has been estimated to be around 50,000, and the majority of those thoughts, let's say 70%, are often negative. When an unhealthy thought or negative vision enters our mind, it's like becoming infected with a debilitating virus that can spread through our brain, to our body, and then to our entire lives. The purpose of this book is to create a healthy environment in our mind so that our positive thoughts can thrive, and then the negative viral ones will be unable to set up camp and multiply. Negative thoughts feed on chaos. If things get a little murky in our mind, then we can catch a cold virus which will run us down for a few days. We can catch the Epstein-Barr virus, best known as "Mono", which will keep us down for a couple of weeks or so. When things get really bad, we can catch a virus that gives us Guillain-Barre syndrome which can paralyze our breathing muscles, slowly and literally taking our breath away. Not thinking well can kill us. Fortunately, the opposite is also true: thinking well can remarkably transform our lives. Can you imagine the effect it would have on your life if you could decrease your negative thinking to 60, 50, or 40% of your thoughts, instead of 70 or 80%?

Sweet Home Chicago

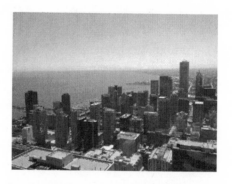

I grew up in a cute and cozy middle class neighborhood of Chicago. Looking back now, my early years seemed magically perfect. I had friends and birthday parties. We went to Florida every summer. But then, as I got a little older, I began to realize that there was something strange going on in my house. No one really spoke to each other; the TV was always on, and everyone seemed to be in their own little world.

My mother never had a job after I was born. She said she was a "housewife" and that's what I should plan on being. I said I wanted to be an actress (inspired by my countless hours of watching TV), but my mother said that was a ridiculous "pipe dream". After her morning chores, Mom would sit in her chair, the one with the worn-out seat cushion, watch her soap operas, and chain smoke all day with the windows closed. In her defense, she had an excuse to not work too hard; when I was around six years old, she had a "nervous breakdown" and the doctor put her on tranquilizers. He told her to take it easy, so that's what she decided to do for the rest of her life. I would sit with her for hours and watch every soap opera, inhaling her secondhand smoke as she blew smoke rings around my head. Then she would make dinner, and my equally amazing father would come home from work. We would all sit around the dinner table in silence as he devoured his food like an angry bear; the only sound you could hear was him grunting and crunching on chicken bones with grease and pieces of chicken splattered all over his face. Then he would watch his news shows in silence for the rest of the night. God knows what my brother did in his room all day; I never really spoke to him that much either. As for me, I was just a lost little girl trying to figure things out, with essentially no help from my family. So the foundation of my preparation for life came from television. I spent my entire childhood watching *Days of Our Lives, The Young and The Restless, Gilligan's Island,* and *The Son of Svengoolie.*

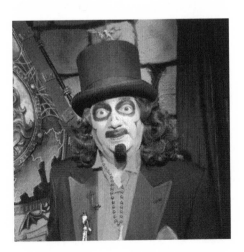

Little did I know, I was about to be unleashed upon the world with almost no tools or skills to handle the dangerous, unchartered waters of growing up. Of course I'm thankful to my parents for the few important life lessons they imparted to me. For example, my father taught me how to go camping, so that came in handy when he kicked me out of the house when I turned eighteen and I had to live in my car. Learning how to go to the bathroom outside is a skill that I had perfected long before I needed it to survive as a homeless person. As for my mother, well, she taught me not to take any crap from anybody. Even though she didn't work or have any friends, and there was no one in her life to take crap from, if anyone showed up with crap, she wouldn't take it!

It wasn't until I reached my early twenties when I came to realize that the model of behavior that my parents presented to me was not the norm, and that the way I was experiencing life was quite distorted as a result of it. I got to the point where depression, anxiety, and fear ruled most of my life, with a few moments of happiness inspired by drugs and alcohol. I knew somehow that things weren't the way they were supposed to be, and that many people really did live calm, happy, inspiring lives with peace at their core, rather than chaos and pain. I wanted so badly to be one of those people, so I embarked on a journey to solve the mystery of how to get a handle on the chaos in my mind, and get the good things out of life that I finally realized I deserved.

*

Fortunately, I have never completely lost my mind, but I often wonder how close I have come. Jeffrey Kluger wrote a fascinating article in *Time Magazine* entitled, *"When Worry Hijacks The Brain"*, in which he vividly describes what it's like to have obsessive compulsive disorder. Reading this article made me feel like Jeffrey was talking about all of us in a way when he said, "Even the most stable brain operates just a millimeter from madness." I have often wondered how close I have come to the edge of oblivion, and it's frightening and fascinating at the same time to think that such a small amount of tissue separates the places in our brain between sanity and insanity. Although the chance of us losing our minds seems remote, it may be more possible than many of us realize, and this is why it's so important for us to improve the quality of our thinking.

Besides not thinking very well, most unhappy people have some other important things in common. They have poor life management skills and poor communication skills, low self-esteem, lack of creativity, poor parenting skills, and probably some sort of mental disorder. According to the Centers for Disease Control, about 25% of US adults have a diagnosable mental illness. That's about 60 million people, or 1 in 4 adults; and 50% of the US population will experience at least one mental illness during their lifetime. So if everyone around you is acting like they're so well put together, they're putting on a good show. How many of these 60 million people have children that they're raising the same dysfunctional way they were raised? We're so worried about which preschool to send our kids to, and how well they're getting to know their fractions, but have we ever once considered if the words coming out of our mouths are going to scar them for the rest of their lives? Are we patting ourselves on the back for being good parents while our children are contemplating suicide? Have we ever explained to our children what "feelings" are? Fortunately, the brain is forgiving, and it's never too late to change it; it's just a little easier if you start early.

*

I must have made some progress, between my twenties and my forties, of increasing my control over the thoughts in my head. Still, I couldn't believe how dissatisfied I was with my life after living it for forty-five years. I had read just about every self-help book out there, and I still kept making the same mistakes. Albert Einstein said that the definition of insanity is doing the same thing over and over again and expecting a different result. This is what I kept doing, and I felt like I was losing my mind. So I started the process of trying to fix my mind all over again, but this time I knew that I had to do something different.

The first thing I did was simplify my understanding of what I was doing wrong, and what I needed to be doing right. Then I drilled what I learned into my head. It was like psychological martial arts, "wax on, wax off", over and over again until it became woven into the very fibers of my being. I started interrogating myself every time I got off track. I would ask myself questions like, "What's making you so anxious?" or, "That was a negative thought, why are you being so judgmental, and what are you afraid of?" Perhaps the most important question that I asked myself was, "What do you want, and what do you need to do to get it?" Then I made myself answer all of these questions honestly and in great detail, and that's when my life really started to change. At first, all of this introspection and life evaluation started making me feel worse. I started having more meltdowns. It seems that I had to come to terms with some of the unpleasant realities of my life that I had been denying or ignoring, and this required going through a little hell before I could make it to the good stuff. Sometimes it's hard to look at yourself in the mirror, which explains why many people refuse to do so. I also learned that I was allowing the chaos in my mind to exist, and this made me realize how much control I really had over my mind. If I could allow the chaos to be there, then I could also refuse to allow it to be there. My only regret is that I didn't figure all this out a little sooner, but better late than never. I also couldn't think of a better way to drill this all into my head than by writing a book about it, and so far it has worked out pretty well for me. Of course, I still have my meltdowns, just not as often as I used to.

*

One of my biggest revelations came when I read Mihaly Csikszentmihalyi's amazing book, *Flow: The Psychology of Optimal Experience*. This book taught me that a gap exists between what we want and what we have, and the quality of our life depends on our ability to close this gap, or to keep it to a minimum, in every moment of our life. I never realized that this "gap" existed, and that the size of it for me, at times, was greater than the Grand Canyon. When the gap is closed, we feel good because we have what we want and there's no conflict. The secret is to maintain this balancing act and keep the gap as closed as possible at all times. From the moment we wake up in the morning, we should start the day by figuring out what it is exactly that we need to do to get ourselves closer to where we want to be.

*

The limits to our potential are psychological, and the purpose of this book is to free our minds from those limitations. Once we take responsibility for being the ones who placed those limitations there in the first place, then we can set about the process of removing them.

14

Once the limitations are removed, the door to the infinite potential of our mind will be unlocked. At the very least, if every little thing we do is geared toward closing the gap between what we want and what we have, we will be increasing our happiness every step of the way. Of course, defining exactly what we need to do to be happier is crucial; we can't close the gap if we don't even know what we want. But we won't be able to get started in the first place if we've never introduced ourselves to the inner workings of our mind.

The ultimate goal is to have more control over our thoughts. So how do we do it, and is it even possible for us *to* do it, since we haven't had much control over our thoughts for most of our lives? The unhelpful ways of thinking and bad habits have been engrained in our brains for 20, 40, or 60 years. I'm not going to start out by telling you that it will be easy to create new and improved pathways for your thoughts to travel over, and to eliminate those deep dark pathways that have already been formed, but it's definitely possible. Besides, *easy* is boring.

Chapter 2

THINK

"As you think, so shall you become"
- Bruce Lee

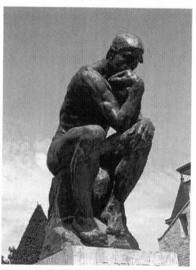

Brain Power

A common belief is that most people use less than ten percent of their brain. While this oftentimes seems true, judging from the lack of common sense that so many people display, the truth is that we use a much larger percentage of our brains all the time, even when we are sleeping or daydreaming. But if we're trying to improve ourselves and improve the way we think, then perhaps asking the question, "How much of our brains are we using?" is the wrong question because it implies a limit to our potential. In other words, if we use our entire brain then that's it; we can't use any more than that. What science and research is beginning to show regarding brain plasticity is that we can create new brain pathways and new connections between brain cells, so the number of new connections that we can make is potentially infinite.

When Albert Einstein died, his doctor removed his brain, sliced it up, and gave pieces of it to the greatest scientists of the day. What they found was that it was about the same size and weight as an average brain. But looking inside, they discovered that the number and concentration of brain cells and connections in certain areas of his brain were far greater than the average brain. So a better question to ask might be, "How much of our brains are we building?"

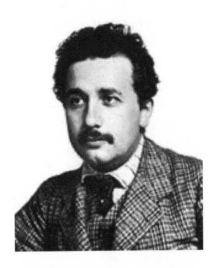

It seems to me that most people aren't building up their brains very much at all. In fact, if we look at a series of brain scans as people age, most people's brains shrink progressively more and more in large part due to abuse and lack of use. Over the past twenty years working in critical care, I've read hundreds of brain scan reports of people over seventy years old and most have the following statement in the report: "atrophy appropriate for age", which means that the scientific community has accepted the shrinking of our brains as a natural and normal phenomenon. But it doesn't have to be this way because much of this shrinkage is due to neglect. The old saying is true, "If you don't use it, you lose it", and this is no more accurate than with the brain. So in order to preserve our brain, we must understand how our mind works. Understanding how our mind works will allow us to control our mind and use our brain more efficiently.

Learning to control our mind is like training a new puppy. Most people don't train their dogs. I see them walking their dogs down the street while the dogs are dragging them along, pulling, jumping, and peeing on everything, while they stand by helplessly throwing their hands up in the air and shrugging their shoulders as if to say, "Can you believe this dog?" Our thoughts do the same thing, and without the proper training, they will be all over the place.

First, we need to define the *mind* so that we can start to understand what we're dealing with. You would *think* this would be easy to do, so easy that no one really thinks about it because they think they already know. The truth is that there are many different theories on how to define the mind, which are all part of one of the greatest debates and unsolved mysteries of science and philosophy. This debate encompasses the most renown scientists and philosophers that have ever lived, including Albert Einstein. Trying to understand and tie together these definitions is like trying to bridge the gap between quantum physics and Einstein's Special Theory of Relativity; ironically, this is exactly what we're going to try and do. But before we talk about that, first we must understand the framework in our head.

The mind consists of our abilities to think and be conscious. To *think* means to ponder the details of something rationally in one's mind. The thinking part of your mind is the analytical part, the part that breaks things down, step by step, adding, subtracting, and figuring it all out. *Consciousness* is the state of being aware - aware of something within yourself or outside of yourself; it allows you to feel the wind blowing through your hair and the sun shining on your face. It also allows you to feel the knot in your stomach when you know your wife is having an affair on you, or when you're engrossed in some complex problem and your conscious awareness notices how quiet your three-year-old is

---

18

being in the next room, it sends you a message that perhaps something might be wrong and you should go check on them.

Some people are good "thinkers". They can answer most of the questions on Jeopardy, and they can tell you off the top of their head how to convert Fahrenheit to Celsius; but their wife walked out on them one day and they don't have the faintest idea why. On the other hand, some people are really conscious of their feelings, but they don't think very well otherwise. These people can tell me how they feel until the cows come home, but if they can't balance the checkbook, it's not going to work. So thinking and being conscious work well together, but not that well alone.

I've spent most of my life thinking that I was a strong thinker. After all, I got really good grades in school and everyone thought I was smart, but I wasn't happy. In fact, I was miserable. Part of the problem was that I wasn't asking myself the right questions, and this is where increased awareness starts. Without asking the right questions, we will be sailing aimlessly towards oblivion.

Know Thyself

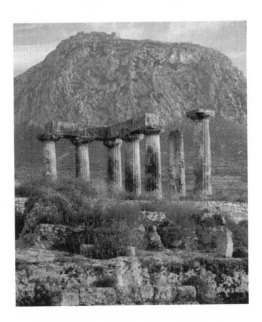

If you want a good lesson on being a strong thinker, you have to go back about 3,500 years to the ancient Greeks. The ancient Greeks figured out that, in order to master their minds, they needed to start by asking the right questions. But if they couldn't figure out the answer to their questions, they would travel hundreds of miles and ask the Oracle of Delphi, who was housed in the great Temple of Apollo.

*

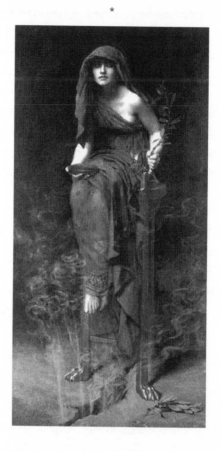

The Oracle of Delphi was called the Pythia, and people came from all over the world to ask her questions about the past, present, and future. The woman who was chosen to be the Pythia had to be an innocent older peasant from the city, and as the presence of the Oracle existed for hundreds of years, many different women played the role. It was believed that the mythical god Apollo spoke through the Pythia, who sat on a tripod seat over an opening in the earth that probably had toxic gases spewing out of it from a fault line that ran through the city.

According to legend, when Apollo killed a Python, its body fell into this fissure and fumes arose from its decomposing body. Intoxicated by the vapors, the Pythia would fall into a trance, allowing Apollo to possess her spirit and give prophesies to those who asked her questions.

As the gases put the Pythia into a trance, she would convulse with incomprehensible speech that could only be translated by the priests of the temple. People consulted the Oracle on everything from when a farmer should plant his crops, to kings asking about the fate of their kingdoms. The Oracle's answers were often given in the form of confusing riddles that were difficult to interpret. A good example was in 547 B.C. when Croesus, the King of Lydia, was considering waging war against the Persians. The king asked the Oracle if it would be wise to go to war, and the Oracle answered that if Croesus attacked the Persians, he would "destroy a great empire". This is one of the most famous statements that the Oracle made, because once the king went to war with the Persians, it became clear that the great empire Croesus was about to destroy was his own.

The famous statement that was carved into the top of the entrance to the Temple of Apollo where the Pythia presented her prophesies was "know thyself", and perhaps the Oracle's main purpose was to get people to think for themselves, by giving them confusing riddles that had to be unraveled, rather than handing people their answers on a silver platter.

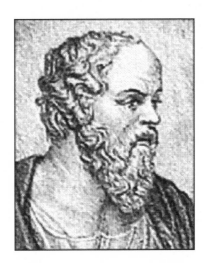

The most amazing person who spent his life *knowing himself* was Socrates, who famously said that "the unexamined life is not worth living." Socrates was alive during the time of the Oracle of Delphi and there's an interesting story involving both of them. It is described in one of the best books written about Socrates, *Socrates' Way: Seven Keys to Using Your Mind to The Utmost,* by Ronald Gross. As the story goes, one of Socrates' friends thought that Socrates was the wisest man in all of Athens, and he sought to prove this by making the journey to Delphi to ask the Oracle, "Is there any man wiser than Socrates?" The priestess replied, "There is no man wiser than Socrates." Socrates didn't understand the Oracle's riddle, because he certainly didn't think he was the wisest man in all of Athens, so he set out to disprove the Oracle. He went to speak to all of the wisest men he knew of, men who surely were wiser than he was. Socrates began to realize though, after questioning these men at great length, that they all thought they were very wise, but at their core they knew very little. Socrates was unable to find anyone that, like himself, was aware of his own ignorance. He ultimately concluded that the Oracle was right; he *was* the wisest man in Athens, because he was the only man who knew that he really knew nothing.

> Happy is he who knows that he knows nothing, or next to nothing, and holds his opinions like a bouquet of flowers in his hand, that sheds its fragrance everywhere, and which he is willing to exchange at any moment for one fairer and more sweet, instead of strapping them on like an armor of steel and thrusting with his lance those who do not accept his notions.
> -Francis Willard

Socrates was one of the wisest people that ever lived because he was able to approach every problem, every question, and every situation as if he was a beginner. Then, by dissecting issues with his mind, he was able to uncover the truth. Unfortunately, the process of uncovering the truth often involves proving other people wrong, and many people don't like admitting they're wrong, especially in public. In the end, Socrates' beloved people, the Athenians, sentenced him to death by poisoning for "poisoning" the minds of others with his ideas. I'm not sure if his beliefs were worth dying for though, so it's important to ask yourself, "do you want to be right, or do you want to be *dead right*?" In any case, Socrates was able to control his thinking and live consciously by mastering the art of asking the right questions.

The Socratic Method

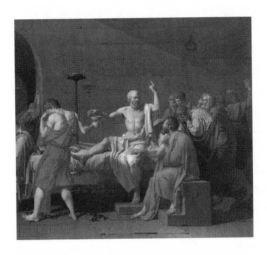

The answer to all of life's problems could be sitting on a platter right in front of your face, but if you don't ask the right questions, you'll never get it. One of the best ways to learn how to ask the right questions is by studying the Socratic Method. The Socratic Method is a process of questioning used by many law schools in the United States to teach their students how to win court cases. Not only can this process be used as a teaching method, it can also be used to deconstruct someone else's position in an attempt to get them to realize that there's a better way to see the situation.

The ultimate goal when using the Socratic Method is to uncover the truth by asking focused questions and periodically summarizing the progress being made, until finally the ultimate truth is revealed. Keep in mind that the wrong questions will lead you in the wrong direction, and the right questions will lead you in the right direction. It's kind of like playing Marco Polo or the hotter/colder game. If your questions are leading you in the right direction, then the answers start to make more sense, and you can feel that you're on the right track. If you're asking someone else the questions though, be aware that some people may not appreciate you picking at them. Socrates was often referred to as a gadfly, a fly that annoys horses and other animals, because he was constantly picking at them with his questions, and we all know how this worked out for Socrates. The problem is that many people don't want to be led to the truth; they're in denial and want to stay there, so you trying to pull them out of their ignorance will be like dragging a hibernating bear out of its cave in the middle of winter. Buttering up your line of questioning by casting a positive light on the other person is always helpful. I like to preface my questions with, "I'd like to ask you a few questions, because I really want to understand your position"; this puffs them up a little before they get deflated.

Just like Socrates conducted his debates with other people thousands of years ago, the Socratic Method enables us to examine common beliefs, and then challenge their validity with other less popular beliefs to reveal a more interesting way of looking at things. This process shines a light where most people either don't want to look, or wouldn't have considered looking. Of course, we're not trying to win a court case here, although some people act like that when they talk to other people. Most people are merely trying to successfully communicate with another human being, and the Socratic Method can make it easier to do this.

The best place to start with this process is to assume that everyone is smarter than you are, and that they have more information than you do. This is so important because, even though it's hard to admit that you don't know it all, often the person you're talking to does have more information than you do. If you approach the conversation as a *know-it-all*, then no one will want to talk to you, because no one wants your opinions crammed down their throat. This position also avoids the embarrassment of acting like you're right when you're really wrong. I've lost count of how many times I thought I was right about something when someone else was questioning my position. Each time, I was unable to resist the urge to tell these people how much experience I had in this area, and that they shouldn't be questioning me. Then I would find out I was wrong and would have to eat my shoe.

The Socratic Method works especially well when dealing with difficult people. In my line of work, I have to deal with difficult people all the time, and I have never been very good at it. But now I know that asking the right questions is the key to dealing with these people. I learned from Ronald Gross, author of *Socrates' Way*, that one of the best things to say to an upset or difficult person is to nicely ask them what they want me to do to make things better. If I can manage to be pleasant and ask them this question despite wanting to strangle them, it always stops them in their tracks because many people have no idea what they want. They're often at a loss for words because they're so fixated on the problem and being negative; it forces them to make the situation positive by searching for a solution.

*

Socrates inspired others to be the best that they can be by teaching them how to think better. Thinking better and constantly reminding ourselves of our own ignorance will lead to an increase in our awareness. But we must also be aware of what's going on around us and how we are affecting the people in our lives. We're not trying to destroy our opponent or win a debate, we're trying to improve the quality of our lives, as well as those around us, and this takes an awareness of how we're affecting other people.

Ignorance means "lack of knowledge", and while most of us think we are experts, we know very little. The problem is that *experts* have so much information crammed in their heads about what they think they know, there's no more room for anything new. I think I'm an expert at many things because I've spent so much time researching stuff, and every day my five-year-old daughter reminds me of my own ignorance. I'll often have a minor, seemingly unsolvable problem that my daughter instantly figures out a solution for, after I've already reprimanded her for disrupting my brilliant train of thought. She can automatically see the simplicity of the solution because her mind is so free, clear, and open to new possibilities. The bottom line is that it doesn't matter how much we think we know, in order to further our understanding, we must empty our minds to make room for new information and better ways of doing things.

By humbly embracing our own ignorance, the path to the truth will be revealed, which will ultimately lead to growth of the Self. We're trying to create the best environment for making a quantum leap with our minds, and being a mature and disciplined thinker, yet having a child-like humbleness and openness to life, will help us do just that. Many people however, are immature, impulsive, and are stuck in a childhood phase of development.

Chapter 3

EGO

In order to better figure out what's going on inside our heads, it will be helpful to refresh ourselves with Freud's structural model of the mind: The *id*, the *ego*, and the *superego*. The path to becoming a mastermind is paved by a well-developed ego. A common misconception is that people who are full of themselves have big egos, hence the words egotistical and egocentric. The truth is that these people have poorly developed and dysfunctional egos, and perhaps it would be more accurate to say that they have small egos, or weak egos. The causes of many psychiatric disorders, especially anxiety disorders, are rooted deep within the dysfunctions of the ego; so if we want to master our minds, we must have a strong and well-functioning ego.

The ego can best be understood by its relationship with the id and the superego. The *id* acts according to the pleasure principle and immediate gratification is its top priority. Like a child, the id is ruled by its own internal desires and has total disregard for the external demands of reality. Freud considered the id to be an unconscious powerhouse of desires that, if left unchecked, would leave us acting impulsively and irrationally. We would take things that weren't ours, touch people we wanted to touch, and say things we wanted to say, without considering the consequences of our actions.

The pleasure principle drives the id to seek pleasure and avoid pain. A child's behavior is ruled by the pleasure principle which is normal at this stage of life, but people stuck at this stage only seek immediate gratification throughout their entire lives, aiming to satisfy all of their internal cravings such as food, alcohol, gambling, drugs, sex, and drama. Look around and you'll have no trouble spotting those people who have never grown out of this stage successfully.

At the other end of the spectrum is the *superego*, which acts as an opposing force to the id. It is associated with our conscience, and its goal is to please the dictates of external reality with socially appropriate and moral behavior. The superego continuously reminds us of what is right and wrong, and punishes us with guilt if we step out of line. The building blocks of the superego were laid by the styles of teaching and discipline of our parents. Having overly strict parents can cause our superegos to become overactive, with guilt and fear filling the center of our lives. Conversely, having parents with a lax disciplinary style can leave us with an underdeveloped superego and difficulty anticipating the consequences of our actions.

Last but not least, this brings us to the *ego*. The ego is the captain of the ship, and its main goal is to balance the wishes and desires of the internal world of the id and the external world of the superego. There is a constant tug-of-war going on between all three of these forces, but the strength of the ego will determine whether or not the ship stays afloat and headed in the right direction.

The ego's job is to please the id with the superego's approval, creating a win-win situation for all and eliminating any conflicts. The problem is that the strength of the id is often greater than that of the ego, so how can the ego control the id? In a famous analogy regarding the ego's relationship to the id, Freud said that, "The ego is like a man on horseback, who has to hold in check the superior strength of the horse." If it is not well developed, the ego will find it difficult to balance the overwhelming drives of the id and the overbearing superego. Without good balance, the scales are often tipped in one direction or the other, with perhaps impulsive addiction on one end, and paranoid or guilt-driven neurosis on the other end.

Not to blame everything on our parents, but it's crucial to understand the impact of parenting on the development of a child's ego. Children will incorporate their parents' ability to maintain balance into their own ego development. The successful parents will have toolboxes full of healthy defense mechanisms to maintain order between the id, the ego, and the superego. I've always assumed that all defense mechanisms are bad, but apparently there are some good ones. For example, using humor to express unpleasant feelings or to deal with a stressful situation is a good defense mechanism. Using the energy from being angry at someone to do something more productive and acceptable, rather than hitting them, is an example of sublimation, which is another helpful defense mechanism. Using the energy from our strong sexual desires and putting it into creating something beautiful, amazing, and useful, rather than developing a sexual addiction, is also a form of sublimation. On the other hand, denial, distortion, and projection are immature and usually destructive defense mechanisms. We need to understand that a lot of what's going on here is unconscious and out of our awareness, so the more we increase our awareness, the more we'll be able to sharpen our good defenses and identify and eliminate the bad ones.

*

Once we understand the basic definition of the ego, it's easy to spot one of its many dysfunctional attributes such as fear, anxiety, narcissism, and addictions to drugs or even drama to name just a few. We're all familiar with the drama queens, those people who infuse every interaction with endless drama, possibly due to an overactive id, making them totally absorbed in the drama of their lives, or the lives of everyone else around them. The drama is like crack to them. Then there are the *Debbie Downers* who, with an overactive superego, find negativity and moral transgressions in everything and everyone. They keep the wheel of conflict continuously turning. If there are problems with these people, the goal is never to find a solution because that would require too much work; the goal is to agitate and perpetuate the problems. Sometimes they put the problems on the back burner and let them simmer for a while so they can turn into even bigger problems. It's perfect; as long as they're totally wrapped up in the drama, they'll never have any time to do anything constructive with their lives because there's always more drama. They'll say, "Oh, I don't have enough time to exercise because I have to deal with this drama!" or, "I don't have time to cook a healthy meal because dealing with the drama took all of my time." If the drama starts to dry up, they go looking for more; or they just watch more of it on TV.

An overactive id requires a continuous stream of immediate gratification, and the source of this gratification can come from many different places. Addictions to TV, video games, drugs, alcohol, and even work are some other examples. A dysfunctional ego can also make people scared and insecure. While they continuously wait for something bad to happen, they remind themselves that there's a good chance they won't be able to handle it when it does.

Another common characteristic of a poorly developed ego is being obsessed with yourself at the expense of others. Like a child that is still ruled by the id, these people are preoccupied with their own internal world, and often have an inability to see another person's point of view. Egocentrism, or perhaps it should be called id-centrism, is the hallmark of early childhood, which is the only time when it's normal to be this way. The problem is that many people never grow out of this stage and remain stuck there for the rest of their lives.

Narcissism

The best picture one can paint of a dysfunctional ego is that of the narcissist. If it's all about anyone, it's all about the narcissist, and the id is ruling the roost with these people. Narcissists are famous for placing their needs above everyone else's. In other words, if the airplane is on fire, they're the first ones out the emergency exit, knocking everyone else over with all of their luggage that they refused to leave behind. Many people are narcissistic, but far fewer people have narcissistic personality disorder. I will be talking about narcissism in general, but it's important to understand the distinction; a much greater degree of narcissism is required to qualify as having the personality disorder.

My favorite subject in school was personality disorders, partly because I thought I may have had a few of them myself, and partly because so many other people seem to have them as well. According to a science update by the National Institutes of Health, about 9% of adults have a personality disorder as defined by the Diagnostic and Statistical Manual of Mental Disorders; 9% of the U.S. population is almost 30 million people, and probably more including the people who've been missed. A study published in the Archives of Psychiatry, which was based on over 5,000 interviews with 19 to 25-year-olds, found that 20%, or 1 in 5 young Americans has a personality disorder.

I think Personality disorders are so fascinating that I've read the Diagnostic Statistical Manual of Mental Disorders just for fun. Once I learned the basic characteristics of all the different personality disorders, I developed an appreciation for how dysfunctional our minds can be. By far, the most fascinating person with a personality disorder is the narcissist. While these people appear stoic, confident, and cool on the outside, and are convinced that they're the most amazing people in the world, they completely unravel when things don't go their way. Ironically, they can also be very hard and critical on themselves.

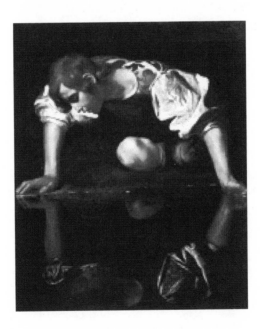

There are several ancient versions of the Greek myth of Narcissus, but the one often quoted is the story of Narcissus and Echo by the poet Ovid, written in 8 AD. As the story goes, a beautiful young man named Narcissus was walking in the woods one day when Echo, a mountain nymph, saw him and fell deeply in love. She followed him everywhere.

When Narcissus sensed he was being followed he shouted, "Who's there?" Echo repeated, "Who's there?" She eventually revealed herself to Narcissus and tried to embrace him, but he rejected her advances. Echo was then heartbroken and spent the rest of her life in lonely glens, until nothing but the sound of an echo remained of her. Nemesis, the goddess of revenge, was enraged by this and decided to punish Narcissus. Knowing that because he was so beautiful, he would not be able to resist seeing his own image, she lured him to a pond where he could see his own reflection. He didn't realize it was only his image and fell in love with it. But because he was unable to tear himself away from looking at himself, he ended up dying there at the edge of the pond. The beautiful flower that grew in his place is called the narcissus, or daffodil.

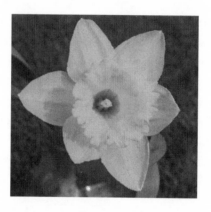

On the surface, it appears that Narcissus had a big ego and loved himself too much; but in reality, Narcissus didn't love himself enough. He wished to possess the person in the reflection who appeared so much more beautiful than he thought himself to be. The irony is that he didn't know the image he was in love with was his own, and he never believed that he himself could be so beautiful. Like Narcissus, so many of us fail to see the beauty within ourselves, and instead search for it, and often think we find it, in others. But just as narcissistic people fail to accept the beauty within themselves and project it onto others, they also can reject unpleasant aspects of themselves and project them onto others as well, as in the case of someone who internally has homosexual impulses but externally expresses prejudice of gay people. The bottom line is that the ego is weak in narcissistic people, creating imbalance and chaos between the opposing forces of the mind.

Whether we'd like to admit it or not, many of us have narcissistic qualities. Much of this can be attributed to our parents not displaying empathy to us and to others when we were young, so we grew up critically lacking empathy ourselves. Lack of empathy is so strongly linked to narcissism because being empathetic requires changing our focus from inside ourselves to the external world of others, something the id would rather not do. Being able to understand and relate to how someone else feels is the key to successful relationships, as well as one of the most important keys to life, which is why narcissists struggle so much in both of these areas.

Some other characteristics of narcissistic personality disorder are an exaggerated sense of self-importance and preoccupation with fantasies of unlimited success, power, beauty, or ideal love. Narcissists require excessive admiration, have a strong sense of entitlement, and are envious of others or believe that others are envious of them. Criticism is poorly tolerated and often responded to with rage, while underneath the rage lies a person with very fragile self-esteem. They also believe they are "special" and can only be understood by other special and high-status people.

Now, I don't want to make this all about me, but when I first read this list twenty years ago I thought, "Oh my God, I have narcissistic personality disorder!" I'm slightly exaggerating here but I did, at one time, possess quite a few of these characteristics, and every now and then, Narcissus rears his beautiful head. I never take advantage of people, but I certainly could be a little more empathetic. I also think I'm pretty "special", and I still suck at taking criticism from others. There's also a survey that psychologists use to assess how narcissistic someone is, called the Narcissistic Personality Inventory. You have to say whether or not you agree with certain statements and my favorite one is, "If I ruled the world it would be a much better place", and to that I still say, "Of course it would be!"

Keep in mind that upon reading the characteristics of all the personality disorders, everyone will find similarities to themselves and other people they know. Someone needs to possess the majority of the criteria listed and display these characteristics most of the time, to a degree that interferes with their relationships and daily functioning, to be clinically diagnosed with the disorder. However, a study published in the Journal of Clinical Psychiatry involving over 34,000 face-to-face interviews in the United States, found that the prevalence of lifetime narcissistic personality disorder was 7.7 percent for men and 4.8 percent for women, a rate that has more than doubled in the last decade. It's also interesting to note that narcissistic personality disorder is placed just below antisocial personality disorder, and many serial killers have antisocial personality disorder. Going back to Jeffrey Kluger's line, "Even the most stable brain operates a millimeter from madness", how much will it take to push someone who has narcissistic personality disorder up to the next level? If our society in general is predisposed to narcissism, what's going to happen now that our children have access to video games that put AK-47s in their hands and encourage them to slaughter everyone in a crowd? I think we're beginning to see the unfortunate answer to that question.

Fortunately though, it's not too late to save our society. So if you or someone you know exhibits some of these characteristics, I found some helpful advice. First, we must be able to recognize those times when we're behaving narcissistically. Becoming more aware of when we're lacking empathy is crucial. The great irony is that what the narcissist lacks in their own character - empathy - is what they crave to get most from others; and since empathy is so difficult to find outside of oneself, the best place to cultivate it is from within. In other words, if we're more empathetic to ourselves, we'll be more empathetic to others. This is why learning some basic "reparenting" skills is so essential to growth. We must treat ourselves like any good parent would treat their child, and fill in the voids that were left from our childhood. If it's discipline that we're lacking, then we need to set some limits for ourselves. If we didn't get enough attention when we were little, then we need to give ourselves some more pats on the back for the accomplishments we've made in life, rather than seeking attention from outside sources. We must give ourselves the empathy that we wish we would have gotten from our parents; we have to tell ourselves that we know how we feel, even if no one else does, and that it's ok to fail. Cutting ourselves some slack will enable us to cut others some slack. It's hard to care how others feel when you're totally self-absorbed, but giving ourselves what we need will allow us to give others what they need.

Having more reasonable expectations of others is also key. Everyone is not going to act the way we think they should, so we need to consider where they're coming from; our way isn't necessarily the best way, or the only way. Working on receiving feedback from others less defensively is, as it was for me, the most difficult thing to do. It's hard to appear grateful when someone criticizes us, but the wise parent inside will remind us that receiving the criticism can make us see things that we weren't aware of before, making us a better person in the process. It's hard, but we can be better by sucking up the criticism, rather than having a temper tantrum. Most importantly, if you think you really do have a personality disorder, you should be talking to licensed therapist.

*

As narcissistic as I used to be, it's ironic how attracted I also used to be to narcissistic people. If you've ever been in a relationship with a narcissistic person, you'll know what I mean when I say that while they're quite entertaining and amusing, they're completely exhausting, and usually over-caffeinated as well, or they're drunk. In any case, each encounter with them leaves you totally drained and wondering, either consciously or subconsciously, what it is exactly that you're getting out of the relationship. This sounds like most of the people I've ever dated, which must have been during the codependent phase of my life. Codependent people love narcissists, because the key characteristic of codependents is that they often place a lower priority on their own needs, while being excessively preoccupied with the needs of others, and who better to be preoccupied with than a narcissist, someone who needs constant attention to feed their weak ego.

It also seems like our society is more narcissistic than any other, considering our generalized self-absorption, fascination with celebrities, and obsession with reality TV shows in which many of us envision ourselves being the star of the show. So we must train ourselves to look past the amazing facade that narcissistic people put up, then we will see how sad and sometimes pathetic these people really are; and we must also never forget how dangerous having a poorly developed ego can potentially be.

*

Narcissism stems from the need to fill a great void, but the void cannot be filled by distractions of immediate gratification and passive pleasure seeking. It can only be filled by reparenting and rebuilding the strength in our ego and our self-esteem. We can't give to others something that we haven't even given to ourselves, and if we don't understand how we feel, how can we understand how others feel?

The moral of the story is that if we accept the good and the bad, and truly love ourselves in a healthy way, we will have confidence in our abilities to make ourselves happy. Then the light of beauty that shines within us will be brighter to us than anyone else's, and we'll know that this inner light will remain within us forever. Wherever we go and no matter what happens to us, it will always be shining. This way, we don't have to remain stuck in one place like Narcissus, trying to hold on to the false view of ourselves or of others. We don't have to cling to something that isn't real for fear of losing it, because you can't lose something that you never had.

Fortunately, in our effort strengthen our egos and become better people, there are many other people who will inspire us along the way - people who have accomplished amazing things despite many obstacles placed before them - people who, before and after their great accomplishments, have remained humble, grateful, unassuming, and not the least bit narcissistic. These people have just the right dose of healthy self-regard that makes them know that they can do amazing things, without hurting other people in the process. These people have well-developed egos, and they have high self-esteem, which makes them capable of transforming something overwhelming into something challenging.

Chapter 4

TOUCHING THE VOID

"Only those who risk going too far can possibly find out
how far one can go" -T. S. Eliot

In contrast to how a narcissistic person is focused only on themselves, focused only on trying to fill the great void at their core - the vast bottomless pit that is forever hungry for admiration and praise and is never satisfied, a secure and successful person has a solid core within themselves that is continuously fed by their own inner light, their healthy love of life and of themselves. This is someone who doesn't fall apart when everything else seems to be doing just that. This is someone who wakes up every morning knowing that, no matter what happens in the course of their day, they can handle it. This is someone like Joe Simpson.

Joe Simpson went through an ordeal that he recounted in his 1988 book, *Touching The Void*, which was turned into one of the best documentaries ever made, and is one of the most amazing and inspiring stories that I've ever heard. It describes the disastrous climb, by Joe Simpson and Simon Yates, of Siula Grande (20,814 feet) in the Peruvian Andes in 1985. They both made it up to the top without a disaster, but on the way down, Simpson fell down the side of an ice cliff and crushed his right leg. After a long struggle, Yates had to cut the rope that Simpson was connected to or they were both going to die. Simpson then plummeted down another cliff and fell into a deep crevasse. Yates, close to death at this point himself, couldn't find Simpson and was convinced he was dead, so he headed back to camp to try and save his own life.

Somehow though, Simpson was still alive, stranded on an ice cliff inside the middle of a huge crevasse, with a broken leg. Even more miraculous was that he was able to get out of the crevasse, barely alive, and crawl and hop over five miles to get back to base camp. He did this all over a three-day period with a broken leg, no food, barely any water, by crawling and dragging himself over the glacier that had more gigantic crevasses scattered all over it.

In the middle of the night, cold and alone, sitting in the belly of a crevasse and already close to death, many people – convinced of their inevitable demise - would have just given up. But what Joe Simpson had at his core was something many people don't: an optimism that can overcome certain death. In order to reach the level of optimism that ultimately saved Joe's life, he had to first accept his circumstances and stop trying to resist the reality of his situation. Joe surely thought that at some point he was going to die there, and he definitely knew that no one was coming to save him. In releasing his grip on the situation and "letting go" in a sense, a bit of relief must have set in knowing that things could not get any worse than they already were. He knew what to expect, there was no mystery about it. Letting himself relax a little about his situation may have led Joe to another thing that sets people like him so distinctly apart from people who give up: accepting his fate as sealed was probably boring to Joe's brain; it was too easy. Perhaps Joe's brain needed a mystery to solve; it needed something constructive to do, rather than just giving up, writing a good-bye note to his family, and waiting to die.

Perhaps Joe's optimism shrugged its shoulders at certain death, and then maybe Joe asked the right question, "Even though it seems like my only option is to just sit here and die, what if I could survive this, and how would I do it?" Once he asked this question, did the universe of knowledge, which his mind somehow had access to, collapse at that moment into the answer that was staring him right in the face? You'll have to watch the documentary to see exactly what happens, but Joe surely knew he was either going to get out of there, or die trying, when many people would have just given up.

Listening to Joe explain his ordeal was one of the most inspiring things I've ever experienced. At times he was often matter of fact about his strategy for making it back, like once he made it out of the crevasse, dragging himself five miles back to base camp wasn't going to be a big deal with a broken leg. His optimism was overwhelming. People like Joe must have been influenced by some very special people in their life that taught them that being positive is priceless. Putting a positive twist on working their way through every obstacle of life is automatic for these people, unlike so many people who are unable to talk themselves into just getting off the couch.

One thing that Joe did to get himself back was to simply break the whole trek into little pieces. He would look for a landmark and say to himself, "If I can just crawl to that next rock," and he would focus on moving just a few feet at a time, with each goal met being an inspiration for the next. Since I've seen this documentary, every time I'm in the middle of a seemingly impossible problem, I picture Joe crawling and dragging himself to the next rock. It always makes what I'm going through seem like a joke compared to what he went through. Joe's strategy for survival is one of the most important ones for overcoming just about any overwhelming challenge in life - breaking it up into small, achievable steps. Trying to conceive of making it back to base camp in his condition must have been unbearable, but he could see the next rock, he could almost reach out and touch it. If every step of our lives is simplified in this way, then anything is possible.

"That which does not kill us makes us stronger"
-Friedrich Nietzsche

Creatively thinking our way out of a deadly situation requires thinking positive. If we want to be successful, then we must remind ourselves that each negative thought that we allow to enter our minds has the potential to set fire to the wooden fortress of life that we have been working so hard to build. While these bad thought processes usually won't cost us our lives in the acute sense of dying on a mountain top, they can result in the slow and painful death of a miserable existence.

Fortunately, for all those *Negative Nancys* out there, having a positive mindset is becoming a popular area of study. Dr. Andrew Weil, in his inspiring book *Spontaneous Happiness,* discusses the field of positive psychology and its chief proponent, Dr. Martin Seligman:

> Seligman observed that those who tend to get depressed following setbacks in life differ from others in how they explain such events to themselves. They take them as confirmation of lack of self-worth, instead of seeing them merely as temporary reversals of fortune. This difference in explanatory styles turns out to be the key difference between optimists and pessimists.

One of the most important things that made Joe Simpson, at his darkest moment, think that he still had a chance was perhaps his ability to control his thinking, and his ability to not let fear and negative thoughts talk himself out of trying to survive. These are the things that have made countless people in history survive such unbearable situations. These abilities are based on a foundation of courage, optimism, and a strong sense of direction. Survivors are guided by an internal compass that always points to living and getting the most out of life.

Chapter 5

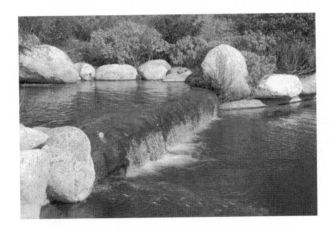

Joe Simpson loved mountain climbing probably because it made him feel better and more amazing than he did when he was doing anything else. Many of us can count on only one hand the few times in our lives when we felt that good, reflecting back on those times as if they were the result of some magical planetary alignment that only occurs every ten thousand years. The truth is that some people are fortunate enough to know how to experience this feeling on a regular basis, without necessarily risking their lives, doing drugs, or becoming addicted to video games. The feeling that we're talking about here is called "flow". But what exactly is flow, and how can we experience it more often?

Simply put, a flow activity is something that we really enjoy doing that is also constructive, productive, challenging, and requires us to learn and develop new skills. Flow has been described as the most amazing experience a person can have because when someone is so absorbed in such an enjoyable activity, no space of consciousness is available to allow unpleasant or irrelevant thoughts to enter.

The concept of flow has been around for thousands of years in many different cultures all over the world, but the first person to describe it in western psychological terms was Mihaly Csikszentmihalyi, who wrote a best-selling book on the subject called *Flow: The Psychology of Optimal Experience.* This is one of the few books that, if you haven't read it, you must; and if you have read it, you should read it again. The specific psychological details that lay the framework for how to achieve this feeling are so effective that they have been used to develop video games, which is one of the main reasons why video games are so addictive: they sadly become more fun than many people have ever had in their real lives. This explains why, according to the Entertainment Software Rating Board, 67% of US households play video games, spending an average of 8 hours per week playing them. The latest study by the CDC states that 41.3% of teens admitted that they played video games or used a computer for something other than school work for three or more hours a day. Even harder to believe is that two books at the top of the current bestseller list are about how to play certain video games, and the latest sales stats show that 273 million video game units were sold last year, leading to 10.5 billion dollars in revenue. Unfortunately, playing video games doesn't usually pay the bills, unless of course the game is actually teaching you something useful, and no offense to the video game industry, but I don't think people who play video games all the time are very cool. I dated someone who did and it was extremely unattractive. In fact, I was embarrassed to admit that the person I was dating played video games at all. Needless to say, the relationship didn't last very long. I would also question how much playing video games contributes to the overall productivity and quality of people's lives. It's great if you learn how to conquer monsters on a deserted island; but if you don't know how to talk to your spouse and children, you get divorced, and your kid attempts suicide because his parents are emotionally unavailable, perhaps you should have been reading a book on mastering your mind rather than playing superhero video games for eight hours a week.

The point is that the makers of these games figured out the formula for getting people hooked without using drugs or alcohol, and that formula is based on getting people into a state of flow. What makes it so profitable for the gaming industry is that most people are unable to achieve this feeling in their otherwise dull and boring everyday lives. The goal is to feel this good actually living your life, not by imagining you're living someone else's.

Can you imagine if most of your waking moments were spent in flow activities that were productive? Let's get a better understanding of this experience so that next time we have it, we'll know it; then we can start reproducing it as much as possible. This is what life is all about.

One of the hallmarks of flow is that all of one's attention is focused on the particular activity that is producing the flow experience. Usually when we do something, we're only using a fraction of our attention because that's all it requires. Most of our daily tasks are preprogrammed. We've been doing the same old job for years, so there's little new challenge there. Many of us get to the point in our lives where we haven't used any more than a fraction of our attention for anything in years, or even decades. We're all walking around like zombies half the time, and since the default setting of the mind is somewhere between chaos at one extreme and apathetic negativity at the other, we spend a good bit of our time just feeling like crap, unless of course you're taking a "feel-good" pill, then you might feel a little bit better than crap, except for the potential side effects of drowsiness, decreased motivation and sex drive, nausea, and anal leakage (just kidding, I don't think anal leakage is a true side effect, but it may be).

So when was the last time you had a flow experience, or seen someone in flow? Sometimes, if you're not in flow and you see someone who is, it's like getting an electrical shock because it makes you realize how far you are from where you should be; or you completely reject their flow and say they're crazy to make yourself feel better about your own mediocre existence. In any case, being in flow is where you want to be, and everyone has to create their own special formula for getting there by defining what they love to do in the finest details.

43

The flow process should make a productive contribution to your life. This generally excludes mindless vacation activities, unless of course you turn them into something that requires learning, brain growth, and challenge; then you get full credit. My family and I take two big vacations every year, one is to a hotel right on the beach and the other is camping in one of our beautiful national parks. The beach vacation costs about $2000 and the camping vacation costs about $150. Now I'm pretty sure that if you took a survey asking which vacation people would choose to go on, most would pick the beach vacation if they could afford it, and no one would argue how beautiful the beach is. For those people who dislike moving too much, the beach vacation is perfect. My partner has a gadget that measures how many steps we take every day, and the beach vacation measured about 3,000 steps daily on average, while the camping vacation measured about 16,000 steps per day. No wonder why most people don't camp.

Trying to achieve a state of flow on the beach vacation is hard for me to do when everything is handed to me on a silver platter. I mean, nothing needs to be done. I don't have to work for anything, and it's just too easy. I struggle to challenge myself mentally and physically on the beach vacation. Now, maybe if I took up surfing I would be more stimulated, but I'm too afraid of getting eaten by a shark after watching that Oprah episode with the girl who got her leg bit off by a shark. Anyway, I would choose the camping vacation every time, and talking about getting more bang for your buck, we could go on ten camping trips for the price of one beach vacation.

We go camping out in the middle of nowhere. There's no running water, no electricity, and no cell phone service; it's awesome! We have a tent and a little travel trailer that keeps our food refrigerated, but besides that, we're living off the land. For me, nothing creates a flow experience better than that. I have a solar panel that I hook up to the trailer to charge the fridge and my computer so I can do some writing. We go hiking and fly kites during the day, and as soon as the sun goes down, the campfire starts and the telescope searches for the rings of Saturn and the moons of Jupiter. When we take a break from the telescope, we see shooting stars and roast marshmallows by the fire, and we talk to each other. The beach vacation is quite relaxing. We sleep, we eat, we lay on the beach, then eat some more, that's pretty much it. Laying on the beach has been glorified on TV and in the movies since the beginning of time, so I think we've been a little brainwashed into believing that it's the best thing ever. Laying on the beach is relaxing, but it's not really that fascinating. Having the light from the rings of Saturn touch my eyeball through the telescope makes my heart skip a beat. Seeing the moons of Jupiter change position each night is mind-boggling. Yes, you have to work a little bit to make it happen, but that's what life is all about, and that's what getting into a state of flow is all about.

Another thing that immediately gets me into a state of flow is building and fixing things. Last summer, I built myself a studio in the backyard to write this book in. It was blood, sweat, and tears; and I loved every second of it. I had to tear myself away from the project to go on vacation; that's when you know you're really doing something you love.

To learn more about getting into a state of flow, you'll have to read Mihaly Csikszentmihalyi's book *Flow: The Psychology of Optimal Experience*. The point of life is to improve the quality of it by getting into flow and trying to stay there as much as possible, but getting to this point is not easy. Simply reading this will not magically turn your life into a Flow experience. You must figure out what it is exactly that you love to do that is challenging, constructive, and brings you great joy. Drugs, alcohol, superficial social contacts, and watching mindless TV doesn't count. If you tell me that you simply cannot find anything else that brings you great joy, then I'll tell you that you didn't try hard enough to find something; and that somewhere along the way, you decided that you just weren't worth the effort.

*

Speaking of being addicted to something, the Surgeon General's latest report on addiction has found that 1 in 7 people will suffer an addiction to drugs or alcohol in their lifetime. Over 47,000 people are now killing themselves each year in the U.S. by overdosing on drugs, with an American dying every 19 minutes from an opioid or heroin overdose. It's too bad that these people didn't have something more important going on in their lives, perhaps their relationship with their children, or an important project that they loved to work on so much that they refused to let drugs or alcohol rob them of the opportunity to finish it. But maybe this wouldn't have been enough to save them. A cruel irony of life is that many of the most amazing people that have ever lived, who were born knowing their purpose and experienced flow throughout their lives, found that it was not enough to save them from themselves. Elvis, Jimmy Hendrix, Janis Joplin, Michael Jackson, Robin Williams, and Prince are just a few on an endless list of people who had flow handed to them on a silver platter and knew their whole lives what would make them happier than anything else, but who also lost it all to the dark abyss of mental chaos and drug addiction.

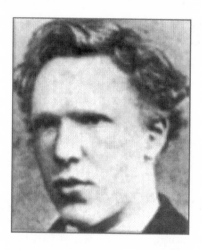

Vincent van Gogh (1853 -1890), one of the greatest artists that ever lived, was one of those people in which flow could not save him from the chaos of his mind, and he allegedly killed himself at age 37. Jeanne Louise Calment's story (1875 - 1997) however, is much different. She was the oldest person to have ever lived on record, living to the age of 122 years and 164 days, and she died in 1997.

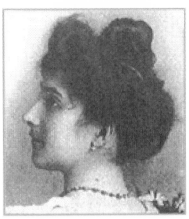

She lived in France her entire life and spent it doing the things that she loved, such as fencing, which she took up at age 85. Jeanne Calment met Vincent van Gogh at the age of 13, when he walked into her father's shop to buy paints in 1888. She remembered him to be "dirty, badly dressed and disagreeable." It's amazing to think that someone who died in 1997 actually met Vincent van Gogh. These two people, whose paths crossed in a brief moment in time, could not have been more different. Painting was the love of Van Gogh's short life, and Jeanne Calment had a few simple hobbies that kept her in flow for over a century. Jeanne Calment figured it out, and Van Gogh never did. No one would argue that this is an unfair comparison because Van Gogh was claimed to be insane by many and Calment had an emotionally stable life. But the point is that achieving a state of flow is not the answer to everything. It is however an essential part of the equation for having a good life, but the more chaos you have in your mind, the harder you're going to have to work to control it.

Chapter 6

HOW FAR WE'VE COME

A good indicator of how well our mind is working, and how well we're controlling the chaos in it, is how often we cry. I'm not sure if I cry more often than the next person, but thanks to my lack of filters, I've always been good at making other people cry. In the words of Johnny Cash, "I taught the weeping will how to cry".

This got me to wonder, how often do people cry on average? The German Society of Ophthalmology, which has examined many different scientific studies on crying, determined that women cry on average between 30 and 64 times a year, and men cry on average between 6 and 17 times per year. Men tend to cry for between two and four minutes, and women cry for about six minutes. This surprised me when I did the math. If you take the low end of how often women cry, 30 times a year, that averages out to about two and a half times a month, or a little more than once every two weeks, and this is the low end? Men on average are crying about once every month or two. This made me think to myself, "Wow, I guess people really aren't that happy." I thought it was bad that I was crying once a week, but it turns out that could be the average for some people.

So where does crying come from anyway? Many theories believe it's an instinct that dates all the way back to the cavemen. Its main purpose could be that of a communication tool, to help reunite lost offspring from their parents, or to allow babies to express when something's wrong because they're unable to speak. It has also been suggested that crying is a way of showing submission to an opponent, or it could simply be used as a way of getting others to help you. Perhaps most interesting is that destructive chemicals and hormones that build up during emotional stress are released in tears, so crying may also serve as a route to eliminate these waste products. This may also be one of the main reasons we feel better after a good cry, because we got rid of these bad chemicals. No study has ever been done to determine the most common cause of crying, but at the top of the list would most likely be a generalized unhappiness and dissatisfaction with life, and an unacceptably large gap between what we have... and what we want.

*

We think that the cavemen probably cried like we do, but the question is, are we any happier than they were? One day in 1994, three explorers were taking a hike in southern France when they accidentally fell into a cave. What they stumbled upon has come to be known as Chauvet Cave, containing possibly the earliest known cave paintings ever discovered, dating to over thirty thousand years old. It was never before apparent that humans had the ability to create cave paintings that long ago, especially with so much detail. They are breathtaking, and present day artists would have trouble reproducing their complexity.

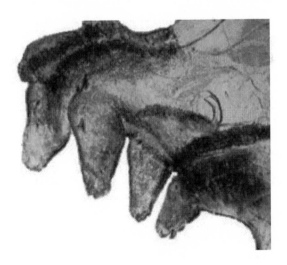

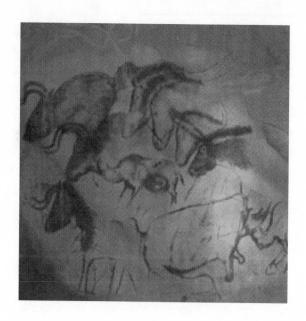

It's fascinating to think of what life must have been like back then, and what people were capable of doing with so much less than we have now. The ability to create such beautiful artwork is a reflection of highly intelligent, fulfilled, and well-rounded human beings who were experiencing flow, possibly more than we do today.

Just try to wrap your mind around a day in the life of a thirty thousand-year-old man or woman. Life was short then, maybe twenty to twenty-five years on average. There was no time to waste. Between hunting and gathering food, fending off mammoth cave bears, and trying to start a fire in the rain by rubbing two wet sticks together, that was their whole day; yet they still found time to create beautiful art. Do you think they had more purpose than we do today?

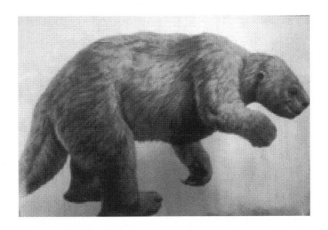

It's a good thing television and video games weren't around back then to eat up all of the cavemens' time; the human species may have never survived. It seems, more so now than ever, that we're spending the vast majority of our time with our faces plastered against the screens of our computers, phones, or televisions. According to the latest Nielsen Cross-Platform Report, the average person watches 4 hours and 39 minutes of television a day. Teenagers are spending an average of 3 hours and 24 minutes a day using a game console. People aged 34-49 are spending an average of 34 hours and 18 minutes a week watching TV; that's another full-time job, if they even have a job in the first place. The last check by the Bureau of Labor Statistics found that almost 91 million people over the age of 16 aren't working in the United States; that's almost 30% of the population, and guess what those people spend most of their time doing? With all of the hours in my life that I've reclaimed from watching TV, I've actually started living my life, rather than watching other people live theirs. Since I've cut my cable cord, I now spend an average of about an hour a week watching TV, and I still don't have enough time to do everything that I want.

Let's do the math here: if you do have a job and work for 8 hours a day, add 2 hours for travel and prep time, then add 4 to 5 hours of watching TV and video games, and sleep for 8 hours, that leaves about an hour left for the most important things in life like face time with your family, friends, and neglected animals. Our TV, video games, phones, and computers have created a huge black hole sucking the life right out of us, while the good stuff is passing us right on by.

It's becoming quite disturbing how distracted we can get with our digital toys in our hands all the time. Some countries have seen a significant increase in the number of toddler drownings. How many of these cases were related to people being too distracted with their digital devices? Recently, a man boarded a crowded commuter train in San Francisco and was shot and killed at random by some crazy guy with a gun. The security footage later revealed that before the gunman fired, he waved his pistol around several times and even rubbed his nose with it, but no one on that crowded train noticed because they were so busy looking at their phones and computers.

While our electronic devices are decreasing our awareness, they are also failing to increase our productivity, as evidenced by the fact that U.S. worker productivity is lower than it's been in decades. It's also quite time-consuming letting ourselves be bombarded with endless amounts of essentially useless information. I've discovered that watching the news religiously, every day for 30 years, has been a waste of time; not to mention how it has traumatized me in the process. It made me want to cry every time I saw the horrible, tragic, and highly disturbing stories that monopolized each news hour. I finally stopped watching the news on TV after they showed a lengthy video of 2 crazy guys covered in blood after they just bludgeoned a British soldier to death on the sidewalk. Previous to that, I had been considering eliminating watching the news from my life because it seemed to be getting more and more disturbing, but I think I was a little addicted to it; it was like seeing a live train wreck every day. Now, I just read the paper; this way I can pick and choose which stories I want to know all the details about, and no more visual trauma for my brain.

The reason we're so addicted to tragic stories, compared to happy and pleasant ones, is because it's in our DNA, and the news producers know it. In other words, this stems from man's beginning as cavemen and how we had to be constantly on guard for threats to our survival. Those who had the quickest and strongest reaction to threats were the most likely to survive. So it's in our genes to have a strong emotional reaction to negative news because it could happen to us; and because so many of us are depressed and scared off the bat, we're convinced that there's a good chance it will happen to us. It's not a question of "if" but "when", we say to ourselves. So we keep watching so that we will be prepared for the onslaught.

Now, instead of watching the news, I spend an extra hour playing games with my family, which is so much more rewarding for all of us. Last year, we briefly turned the news on to watch the coverage of a gunman loose in the mountains that we often visit. After that, our three-year-old daughter was putting up barricades around the living room to keep the bad guys out. Now she's not being traumatized either.

So what would we do without TV and all our digital toys? What would we do without our video games and the internet? Would we draw? Would we learn how to play the guitar? Would we have time to do all the things we said we wanted to do in order to make our lives more complete? Would we cry less? What would happen if we all had so much extra time to think about doing something more productive than watching other people live their lives on TV? Would we be happier than a caveman living thirty thousand years ago? It has been said that human progress is a result of technology freeing us up so we have more time to be creative, to create things that will make life better. Doesn't it seem like technology stopped doing that somewhere along the way? Children aren't being taught handwriting in school, and people don't even know how to talk to each other anymore; is this progress? If we're going to watch TV, we should make sure we're going to learn something constructive from it. When was the last time you learned something new? Sophisticated people in the olden days could speak five languages fluently. Today, people are considered sophisticated if they can speak their own native language well.

Not only have people, and especially children, lost the ability to speak to one another properly, but art and music classes have been eliminated from schools, so they won't even be able to make a cave painting if they wanted to. They also won't be able to write you a letter because handwriting has been eliminated from the curriculum as well. If you have any money to invest, you should buy some famous handwritten documents, because they're becoming even more valuable with the disappearance of anything important actually being written down.

Draft of Gettysburg Address

Having had to read the most illegible handwriting by doctors in medical charts for over two decades has created a special place in my brain for performing such amazing feats. But with the advent of electronic charting, that place is disappearing fast, and it's a shame. People used to come to me all the time to help them decipher the hieroglyphics of doctors handwriting, but not anymore.

An article I found in The Wall Street Journal was talking about a certain grocery store's marketing strategy. The store was considering putting a product on its shelves that had cursive handwriting on the label, but the store insisted that the cursive handwriting be changed to printed lettering. The reason, the store's buyer stated, was because "Millennials can't read cursive." I knew this was a problem, but I had no idea of its global impact. It's official though, there's now an entire generation of people that can't read *or* write cursive.

So, if people end up having some free time on their hands because they put their devices down, one thing they might want to consider doing is writing something down in cursive. They could start a journal that they could one day give to their son or daughter, but that might be too much self-examination to start out with. Maybe they could teach their children the lost art of cursive. They could teach their child how to fly a kite, make a sundial, or just tie a real pair of shoes, rather than velcroing their "special" shoes together. They could take the family camping in a real live tent, out in the wilderness, and teach everyone how to see our neighbor galaxy Andromeda through a pair of binoculars, instead of going on a $2,000 amusement park vacation. I guarantee you that you and your family will be far more inspired by seeing a shooting star through the Milky Way for free.

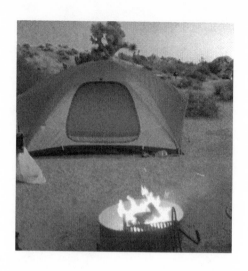

The bottom line is that we may not be happier now than we were fifty, one hundred, and perhaps even thirty thousand years ago. The question is, how do we define quality of life? If someone lived the slaughterous life of a caveman for only twenty years but loved every minute of it, wouldn't they have been happier than someone who lived for eighty years and spent most of it sitting on a couch complaining about how rough they had it? Maybe we just have too much time on our hands now that we don't have to go all the way down to the river to wash our clothes; but it was nice going down to the river, and I have yet to see a study that shows we're any happier than we used to be with all of our new technology. Perhaps we should use the number of people who throw themselves off bridges as a benchmark for how satisfied we are in general as a species. There probably weren't too many cavemen jumping off cliffs thirty thousand years ago, because they were too busy trying to stay alive.

Chapter 7

THE RIGHT STUFF

"Two things are infinite: the universe and human stupidity; and I'm not sure about the universe." -Albert Einstein

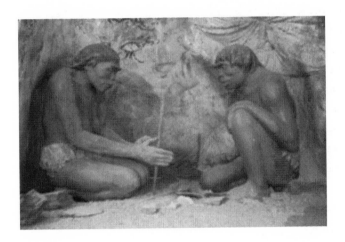

Smarts

So my next question is, are we any smarter than the cavemen? According to a *Discover Magazine* article written by Kathleen McAuliffe, "If Modern Humans Are So Smart, Why Are Our Brains Shrinking?", recent research indicates that in the last 20,000 years, the volume of the human male brain has shrunk about 10% from 1,500 cubic centimeters to 1,350 cubic centimeters. Some researchers think this decrease in size is due to the brain becoming more efficient and thus requiring less energy. But others think it indicates that humans are getting dumber because, with the advances in technology, we don't need to be that smart to stay alive anymore. This is the problem, isn't it? It's too easy for us now. We wake up, we go to work, pay the bills, and drive the kids to soccer practice. We need some challenge and adventure in our lives if we want to stay smart. People are now losing their minds to Alzheimer's Disease at an alarming rate, with it now being the sixth leading cause of death. Women in their sixties now have a greater chance of getting Alzheimer's Disease than breast cancer. Could the answer to the problem be as simple as we're just not using our brains enough? Ironically, third world countries have the lowest rates of Alzheimer's Disease. One theory in the scientific community links this to poor hygiene, stating that these impoverished people's increased exposure to viruses and bacteria makes their immune system stronger which in turn protects their brains. But could their struggle to survive also be making their brains more immune to getting Alzheimer's Disease? Anxiety has also been found to be much lower in less developed countries, based on a World Health Organization survey which found that experiencing anxiety in any one year was 18.2 percent for Americans and 6.8 percent for Mexicans. Nigeria had the lowest levels of anxiety at only 3.3 percent.

As far as why our brains have been shrinking for the last twenty thousand years goes, no one has come to a definitive conclusion; but one thing is for certain, it oftentimes doesn't feel like we're any smarter than the cavemen. So if we want to master our minds, it helps if we're kind of smart.

The standard way of measuring our intelligence has always been the old-fashioned IQ test which mainly measures analytical intelligence. Analytical intelligence measures one's ability to solve problems that are more concrete and usually have just one answer. It helps us analyze, compare, and evaluate all the facts before we come to a conclusion. People with high IQ's do well in school because that's what school is all about: solving analytical problems like math or chemistry equations. I remember when I had my IQ tested in a high school psychology class and I think it was somewhere in the 120s, so I guess I'm not a genius. I haven't had it measured again since, but I'm sure it's a little bit lower now. What I learned back then though is still a surprise to me today, and that is that the average IQ is around 100. If you want to find out what your IQ is, there are several online sites where you can test yourself.

Below you can find the Wechsler classification and what percentages of the population fall into the different IQ levels:

Wechsler Adult Intelligence Scales Classification

IQ Range - Percentage of population

128 and over - Very Superior - 2.2%
120–127 – Superior - 6.7%
111–119 - Bright Normal - 16.1%
91–110 - Average - 50.0%
80–90 - Dull normal - 16.1%
66–79 - Borderline - 6.7%
65 and below - Defective - 2.2%

According to the table, I'm in the superior range, but how come I only feel slightly above average? In fact, I often feel like I'm operating at the defective "imbecile" level, which used to be the label applied to the people scoring the lowest on the scale. Am I really that much smarter than most of the population? I'm certainly not more successful than the average Joe.

People who are considered really smart and win special awards usually have IQs somewhere in the 140s. So does that mean I'm not going to get a Pulitzer Prize for writing this book? Well, not necessarily - don't count me out yet; if Bob Dylan can win a Nobel Prize, maybe I can win something too. A study conducted by J. Robert Baum of the University of Maryland found that regardless of the level of analytical intelligence, those who had a high level of practical intelligence were far more likely to succeed in their business ventures. Baum states that practical intelligence, or "hands-on" learning versus learning from reading or watching, "best reflects abilities that enable entrepreneurs to cope with their extreme situation (high uncertainty, urgency, insufficient personal resources, and rapid change)."

In contrast to analytical intelligence, which we get mostly from book smarts, we get practical intelligence by learning from our experiences and adapting our behavior accordingly. This type of intelligence is often referred to as "street smarts". Robert Sternberg, a leading researcher on human intelligence and also the author of *Practical Intelligence In Everyday Life*, describes practical intelligence as the ability to create a good fit between ourselves and our environment through a three-faceted process of adaptation, shaping, and selection. In other words, when something happens to us, we have three general choices in how we respond to it. First, we can *adapt* to it by changing ourselves to fit the environment. For example, if clouds are forming in the sky we can bring our umbrella. If we see thugs on a street corner, we can turn down another street, and then never go down *that* street again in the future. If someone's comments are bothering us at work or at school, we can choose to ignore them and remind ourselves that we don't care what they think anyway. We can also try to *shape* our environment to better fit us. If it's too cold in the house, we can turn up the heat. If unfavorable conditions are created at our job, we can form a committee to try to make the environment work better for us. Lastly, *selection* is the choice of finding or selecting a completely new and better environment, if all else fails. If we cannot accept the unfavorable conditions at our job, and are unsuccessful in changing them, then we can always just get a new job or a new career. The chaos of life becomes structured and simplified by knowing we have these basic choices; it gives us powerful control over our environment. People who have high levels of practical intelligence are experts at knowing which choice is the best. They're also able to use their practical intelligence to realize when they're on the wrong path in life, so that they can change direction before too much time has been wasted.

By no means am I discounting analytical intelligence. If you have a high IQ, then you're ahead of the game; and although a large part of our analytical intelligence is genetic, there's also another large part that isn't, which means you can improve it. You can always make yourself smarter in a certain area by simply sticking your head in a book and making yourself learn the material. Then you can combine this solid knowledge base with some basic problem solving skills such as identifying the problem, identifying a solution, and figuring out how to get from point A to point B the most efficient way. But analytical intelligence falls short by often being narrowly focused, overly structured, and often devoid of the practical intelligence qualities of creativity, intuition, and common sense; it's a little more challenging to increase these qualities within yourself. You can start by training yourself how to better adapt to, shape, and select your environments. You can combine this with intuitively increasing your awareness of everything, creatively asking the right questions, and learning from your successes as well as your failures.

It's nice to know that there are things we can do to make ourselves just a little bit smarter in whichever area we need to the most. Keep in mind that if your IQ is around 100, you still have a chance to be an amazing person and succeed at great things, and there are plenty of people walking around with IQs in the 140s who really haven't done anything special with their lives.

*

IQ tests weren't around thirty thousand years ago, but one things for sure, the cavemen and cavewomen were smart enough to survive, and they surely lived their lives to the fullest. So it does seem plausible that our brains are shrinking because we don't need to be that smart to stay alive anymore. I wonder how that's effecting the trajectory of the human race? Life expectancy has, for the first time ever, started to shrink for certain parts of our population. Less-educated Caucasians have lost four years since 1990, and Caucasian women without a high-school diploma lost five years. So the more educated we are, the longer we're likely to live.

*

Henry David Thoreau said, "The mass of men lead lives of quiet desperation": same worries, same job, punch in, punch out, same bad jokes. If improving our practical intelligence requires learning from our experiences, we have to start having some experiences; we have to shake our lives up a little bit if we want to prevent our brains from shrinking.

Do something different for a change. How would you spend your life for the next six months if you knew they were your last? The cavemen certainly lived each day as if it was their last; perhaps this was their greatest motivation.

The Allegory of "The Cave"

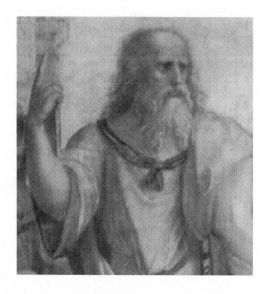

Even though our lives originated in caves, and even though the cavemen may have actually been smarter than us, that doesn't mean we should still live in caves or really have a "cavemen mentality". Plato, whose teacher was none other than Socrates himself, gave us a fascinating example of the differences between smart people and ignorant people with his classic allegory of "The Cave", which was actually a conversation that Socrates had with Plato's brother. Socrates was discussing the differences between unenlightened people who rely solely on the sensations from their body to know reality, and those who are enlightened and use the logic of their mind to ultimately know what is true and real. To illustrate this, he used an example of prisoners chained to a wall inside of a cave. Between the prisoners and the opening of the cave is another short wall, and behind this short wall are people holding up puppets of different things moving back and forth.

Behind the puppets is a fire that casts shadows of the puppets on the wall of the cave. The shadows on the wall are the only things the prisoners ever see, so they assume that the shadows are real things and represent their own true reality. Should one of the prisoners get free, they would look around and realize that the shadows in the cave were not real things, only puppets. They would see the sun shining through the mouth of the cave and follow it outside where they would see real things for the first time. Then they would be able to tell the difference between real things and shadows. Wanting to share this amazing knowledge with their fellow prisoners, they would return to the cave to tell everyone the truth and help free them from their chains of ignorance. The prisoners, out of fear of the unknown, would reject the truth from this messenger, consider them insane, and want to kill them. (Please forgive my horrible drawing below)

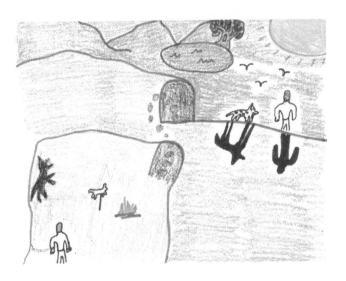

The point is that it's hard to get people to let go of their shadows of misunderstanding, and many would rather take their ignorance to their grave rather than exchanging it for something more rational. The process of mastering our minds is like the allegory of *The Cave* in that we've spent our entire lives, in some cases, living in a cave of ignorance. We let our senses, especially those of hunger and pain, run our lives without really being aware of what's happening. If we feel hungry we immediately eat, because god forbid we let ourselves be hungry for a little while, so we eat and eat and eat, even though we don't need the calories. We've eaten so much that 29% of the global population, or 2.1

billion people, are now overweight or obese. If we move too much and we feel tired, we immediately stop because god forbid we move too much and get too much exercise. If we get a knot in our stomach because we're letting our hopes and dreams slip away, then we take a pill for that, instead of figuring out what our purpose is here. If we have any other pain, we take a pain killer, instead of figuring out what we did wrong with our body and how we can heal it naturally. The Centers for Disease Control states that "the misuse and abuse of prescription painkillers was responsible for more than 475,000 emergency department visits, a number that has nearly doubled in just five years." Not to mention the overdoses:

> In a period of nine months, a tiny Kentucky county of fewer than 12,000 people sees a 53-year-old mother, her 35-year-old son, and seven others die by overdosing on pain medications obtained from pain clinics in Florida. In Utah, a 13-year-old fatally overdoses on oxycodone pills taken from a friend's grandmother. A 20-year-old Boston man dies from an overdose of methadone, only a year after his friend also died from a prescription drug overdose. These are not isolated events. Drug overdose death rates in the United States have more than tripled in the last 2 decades and have never been higher.

When our senses tell us we're in pain, they also tell us to make it go away as soon as we possibly can. Our senses don't care *how* we do it, just as long as we *do* it. The pills take away our pain as they slowly kill us; such is the fate of an unenlightened life. Of course, I'm not talking about the small part of the population that has chronic, intractable pain issues, or is dying of a painful cancer; these people need pain medicine to help them live longer, and I'm not talking about people who need a couple pain pills to get through a temporary operation. I'm talking about everyone else who hasn't bothered to try and figure out why they're in pain, or research how they can make themselves feel better without taking pain pills.

We have imprisoned ourselves in the cave of our own lack of awareness and fear of the unknown. We know it's dark, damp and cold in this cave, but it's been our home for so long, and who knows what's really going on outside of it. It feels safer to stay where we have been; at least we know what to expect here. Fortunately, there will always be a select few who decide to climb out of the cave by expanding their awareness. These people will be the ones who continuously ask all of the right questions that most of us are afraid to ask. It is a rare quality to have the courage to venture into the unknown, and many of these people will have to make that journey alone.

Alone

Another quality of high intelligence is the knowledge and understanding that to truly master something requires spending an extraordinary amount of time learning and practicing it, perhaps as much as 10,000 hours or more, as noted in Malcolm Gladwell's book *Outliers: The Story of Success*. You can do the math yourself to figure out how many years that will take you, but if you're working at it for twenty to forty hours a week, that would be about five to ten years. To spend that much time studying something, learning all of the hundreds and thousands of facts and storing them in your brain, often requires spending a good bit of that time alone. I think it would be safe to say that if you can't stand being alone, you probably won't be very successful at many things, including controlling your thinking.

"An idle mind is the devil's playground"

This quote answers the question of what happens when people suck at being alone - they get into trouble, or they start feeling like crap because negative thoughts flood their minds. In other words, if the mind has nothing structured to do and nothing good to think about, evil thoughts and deeds will take over. Like many things though, the meaning is so obvious that we don't often give it a second thought. But if you could sum up in one line what the biggest problem is for the majority of people on this planet, it could be as simple as - they're bored. Many people just don't have anything constructive to do or think about, and they hate being alone. Trying to stay alive doesn't take the whole day anymore, and if people don't have anything constructive to do, they often resort to destruction. They will either destroy themselves or they will destroy everything around them.

Many people will go to the ends of the earth to avoid being alone. The digital toy and internet companies of the world have capitalized on this, and the irony is that the CEOs of these companies are the ones who have spent countless hours alone, mastering business and information technology, and now they rule the world. One needs to look no further than the astronomical success of social websites to prove this point. To this day, I rarely visit these websites because I'm so busy actually living my life, as opposed to reading about how other people are living their lives, and it amazes me how some people spend most of their time on them.

We must teach our children, as well as ourselves, that learning to enjoy being alone without TV, social websites, or video games, is imperative to achievement and success, and that it can be a great source of enjoyment, rather than pain. I'm not saying people should never indulge in digital distractions, but five hours a day is ridiculous, and strong social ties are very important for our health, but superficial interactions don't really count. Alone time should be sought out, cherished, and cultivated, not wasted or avoided like the plague. With the extra time that we have left over after doing the essentials, clear and structured goals should be considered. I can't remember the last time I didn't have anything to do or think about. I often even turn the radio off in my car because what's going on in my head is so much more interesting and important. On the rare slow days at work, I'm amazed at how many people spend the entire day just talking and going from one person to the next, talking about what they watched on TV, or what they're going to eat at their next meal, or who spent the most time sitting on the couch yesterday sleeping. As soon as one conversation ends, they find someone else to talk to. I can sit for hours just quietly thinking and strategizing my life without ever talking to anyone; maybe those people think *I'm* crazy.

The bottom line is that many of the most successful and amazing people spend the greatest amount of time alone. So if you want to do

---

something amazing, or even if you just want to be a more interesting person, turn everything off, and take a look inside. If you don't enjoy looking inside yourself, chances are, no one else will either.

Other Life Management Skills

*Make yourself look in the mirror, even if you don't like what you see. If you want to improve the quality of your life, you're gonna have to come clean to yourself about your shortcomings. Everyone must realize that when they look in the mirror they may not like everything they see, and that's ok. It doesn't help that everyone on TV and in magazines looks and acts like *genetically-engineered-to-perfection* humans, but we have to remind ourselves that those people are actors with fake appearances, that they don't really look like that in real life, and if we had a team of fifty people working on us for two hours we would look and act that amazing as well. Some people can go for years without ever really looking at their own reflection. Some businesses have even capitalized on this fact by providing exercise facilities that don't have any mirrors. Someone once said, "If looking at yourself in the mirror makes you feel like crap, then this place is for you!" Really, no mirrors when you're working out or lifting weights? That's like painting with invisible paint; what's the point? I mean, I know we're not supposed to be obsessed with our own images like Narcissus, but isn't one of the greatest benefits of exercising improving how we look? We must be more in touch with the real reflection of ourselves so that we can see what we have to work with, rather than fumbling around in the dark.

*Listen to yourself the next time you're complaining about life and ask yourself what it is, if anything, that you could be doing about it.

*Question yourself, and tell yourself the truth when you answer those questions. We have to be honest with ourselves and admit when something isn't working. Recognizing early that we have failed despite making a valiant effort to make something work is key; we have to be willing to cut our losses.

*Take action in your life. Having control over our internal and external lives requires taking action. This goes back to practical intelligence, our relationship with our environment, and the options of adapting to, shaping, or selecting a new environment. If we don't like our jobs, we could get a new one (selection), or change the way we see our current job (adaptation). If we don't like the way our partner is acting, we could try to be more empathetic and consider where they're coming from, or perhaps realize that they're not perfect and accept them for who they are, since we ourselves are surely far from perfect (adaptation). If someone is being disrespectful to us, we could tell them that we won't tolerate their behavior (shaping). The point is that we could DO something about the things that we're dissatisfied with in our lives, we could DO something to decrease the gap between what we want and what we have. Every morning when we wake up, we need to ask ourselves what it is that we should be doing to improve the quality of our lives. The problem is that many people don't like to do anything if they don't have to. After all, they've been doing as little as possible to get by most of their lives, and if they start to do something extra now they'll be opening up a whole new can of worms. I mean they may have to finish what they started, and that could be time consuming, and then they won't have enough time to watch all the shows that they've previously recorded, so maybe they shouldn't even bother. Turn everything off and get off the couch.

*If you do decide to get off the couch and actually do something with your life, an indispensable tool to use is priming. As a fuel injector primes a car's engine with gas so it can fire up as soon as you turn the key, priming our minds with exactly what we're going to do before we do it allows us to lunge out of the starting gate, while others who haven't primed themselves just stumble around for a while before they really get going. This works quite well with children too. I always review the plans for the day with our daughter so she knows what to expect.

*Embrace failure. One of my favorite lines was spoken by Hillary Clinton when an interviewer asked her what her secret to life was and she said it was her ability to "embrace failure". Thomas Edison once said that he had to succeed because he ran out of things that wouldn't work. Failure is a gift from the gods, and our journey here will be made so much easier if we can somehow get ourselves to view it this way. Embracing failure requires us to learn from our mistakes so we do not repeat them. Many people spend their entire lives running over the same ground by making the same mistakes over and over again, because they are somehow able to forget that what they keep doing isn't working.

"Those who don't remember history are destined to repeat it"
-George Santayana

Chapter 8

MISERY IS OPTIONAL

I have been wrestling with anxiety for a good portion of my life, and have often wondered if it would be easier if I was taking something for it. Fortunately, my nursing background has given me a detailed understanding of how drugs work, as well as how the body works, so I've been able to make a more informed decision about whether or not to take medication for my anxiety. I know how powerful the brain and body can be under the right circumstances, and I think that many people who take medication off the bat underestimate this power, so they end up overvaluing the pills and undervaluing their own capabilities. My mother is one of those people who has underestimated her own power, and as a result has been on several psych meds for most of her adult life. As a child, I had to sit by and helplessly watch the marrow slowly seep out of her life because she was overmedicated for most of it. She was bounced around from one doctor to the next, with each one adding another medication to her regimen, because no one could make her happy in fifteen minutes, so giving her another pill was the easiest thing to do.

Despite all of the medication that she has taken, my mother has been pretty unhappy for most of her life. It seemed that all the medication did was to get her to pipe down a little bit and not get so riled up, but it never got her to think better. So I'm not a big fan of taking any kind of medication unless it's absolutely necessary. Not that these medications don't help countless numbers of people who are still miserable despite having tried non-drug remedies, or those who are in danger of hurting themselves or other people, but I'm not convinced that my mother really needed them because she never really tried to make herself feel better without the drugs, so we'll never know for sure. As for myself, I've been bound and determined to do everything I can to avoid taking any pills, but I have come close a few times. It's hard being the only one who gets riled up about stuff when everyone around me is so calm.

While I was trying so hard to feel better on my own, it seemed like everyone else was just popping different pills and bragging about how great they felt on the medication. Then I came to realize that many of these people really hadn't changed, and they really didn't seem any happier than they were before; they never got their stuff together, and they seemed less focused. If they didn't have any goals or hobbies before, they still didn't. The people who were overweight were still overweight, and they were still constantly cramming bad food in their mouths all day long while they complained about not ever being able to lose any weight no matter what they did, even though they weren't really doing anything. If they hated their jobs before they took the pills, they still hated their jobs. If they had trouble sticking up for themselves when they were being taken advantage of, they still bit their tongues instead of saying what was on their minds, and if they had a history of being in bad relationships, they were still dating losers. I wondered if all the medication did was to make the mirror they peered into everyday reflect back a less focused view, so that it would be easier to look at themselves. Let me be clear, I'm not talking about the people who are clinically depressed, or whose anxiety is making it difficult for them to perform their daily activities, or the people who want to jump off a bridge. There are a significant number of people who do need to be medicated, and if you're one of them then for the love of God, don't let me stop you. For everyone else, if you've done everything to try to make yourself whole - if you're exercising every day, writing a journal, eating healthy, and talking to a therapist and you still feel like crap all the time then perhaps you should be on something, and maybe you will feel better then. Maybe I'm the idiot who's killing myself trying to feel better on my own without medication; I've certainly had my moments of doubt. But I haven't let those moments of doubt define me or take me over. Everybody feels like crap sometimes, and I'm dealing with those times a lot better than I used to. I'm proud of all the work I've done on myself, and if I was numb to the pain I was feeling then I never would have done all this work in the first place, there would have been no need to. The pain is there for a reason.

*

In my late teens, after my parents got divorced, things started to unravel for me. I was homeless, jobless, friendless, and very depressed. I was terrified that, like my mother, I wouldn't be able to take care of myself. So I decided to get the best paying job with the most job security I could find. That job turned out to be in nursing. I ended up going into critical care, and have been an intensive care nurse for the last twenty years. The only problem was that I didn't really like being exposed to blood, vomit, and feces on a daily basis, with people yelling and screaming at me, alarms going off constantly, and people dying, ugh! What was I thinking? What I didn't know when I started my career was that I had an anxiety disorder, and that doing one of the most stressful jobs around was not going to be the best idea for me. So writing this book has been quite helpful in dealing with my job, among other things.

Quite often, being an ICU nurse is like living inside of a horror movie. A good number of patients are confused, withdrawing from drugs or alcohol, or just plain out of their minds. The other day, a patient got confused, pull all his IVs out, ripped off his clothes, and came walking up to me at the nurse's station covered in blood and screaming; it is, at times, a living nightmare. Another time, a confused patient called the police and said we were trying to kill her, and we had to convince the 911 operator that we really weren't trying to kill the patient, even though we wanted to (just kidding). Then there was that time when a confused patient tried to strangle my coworker and we had to call the police to come and get control of him, or when my combative patient punched me in the face and broke my glasses. Of course, it's not always this dramatic, just frustrating, like when I get my patient all neat and tidy and then they projectile vomit and diarrhea all over everything, and there's no one to help me clean it up.

Don't get me wrong, I'm very thankful for my job, and I've had a lot of amazing experiences. Working in critical care gives me the elite privilege of saving people's lives, and it's amazing to think that there are many people out there that wouldn't be alive today if it wasn't for me. Most people can't brag about that, but the problem is that it's quite unpleasant. My advice to you is, figure out what makes you the happiest, and spend most of your time doing it. My other advice to you is, don't get sick. If chaos is in your mind, it will be in your heart and body, and you will get sick, I guarantee it.

Anxiety

"What you resist will persist"
-Carl Jung

Anxiety, fear, and anger are all fruits from the same kind of tree, and the dish we make with them is called misery. To begin to understand this, we must go back to our old friends, the cavemen, and remember that these primal emotions kept us alive when we were being chased down by woolly mammoths, but they're not woolly mammoths anymore, they're our bosses, co-workers, or perhaps even our spouses. These overwhelming responses aren't usually necessary anymore, but they're still there.

Anxiety disorders are broken down into generalized anxiety disorder, obsessive compulsive disorder, post-traumatic stress disorder, and phobias. The National Institutes of Health has found that approximately 40 million American adults, or about 18.1% of people in this age group, have an anxiety disorder in a given year. Generalized anxiety disorder is characterized by persistent worrying and tension that interferes with day-to-day activities. The course is usually a chronic waxing and waning of symptoms such as tightness in the chest, knot in the stomach, increased heart rate with palpitations, irritability, and negative thoughts. When I first wrote out this list of symptoms, I realized that this is exactly how I used to feel each time I went to work at the hospital.

One of the main problems that people with anxiety disorders have is something called "errors in logic", which is another way of saying that they don't think well. These are distorted patterns of thought that cause us to negatively and inaccurately perceive reality. The pathways that these thoughts travel over were laid down years or even decades ago, and our thoughts keep traveling over them, again and again. Here are some examples of these errors in logic:

*Selective abstraction involves only giving negative thoughts and events credit while disqualifying the positive ones; I used to do this all the time - if something good happened to me then it was an accident, and I would automatically think something bad was going to happen soon to make up for it.

*Always assuming the worst or catastrophizing: this one's my favorite. I would assume that every outcome would be a worst-case scenario. If someone was late, then I'd think that they must have died in a car accident. If I found a new mole on my leg, I would automatically assume it was cancer and that I was going to die. If I found a little water in the boat, then the whole ship was going down.

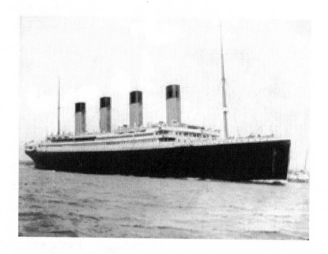

*Unrealistic expectations: another one of my favorites - thinking other people should behave like I do without considering where they're coming from, or thinking that my way is the best way to do something. Expecting everything to be perfect and that nothing will go wrong is also totally unrealistic.

*Dichotomous thinking is viewing things or people as all good or all bad, when in reality there's usually a large grey area in the middle that needs to be considered.

Working to decrease our errors in logic will help ease the pain of many things, including going to a job that we dislike. But if we still don't like it, then no amount of "thinking well" will change that. We can change our thinking and lower our expectations, but if these two things don't work then it's time to select a new environment.

Social Anxiety

One of the most common types of anxiety is social anxiety. Social Anxiety is described as an uncomfortable feeling that is experienced in social interactions when someone is fearful of being judged or evaluated by others. People with social anxiety are concerned about being embarrassed, criticized, or rejected in some way by their peers. This is related to low self-esteem in that they lack the confidence in their ability to speak or perform in front of others. Developmental social anxiety occurs in early childhood, is a normal part of social development, and most children grow out of it. Those who don't, however, go on to develop chronic social anxiety.

The role that low self-esteem plays in social anxiety is related to how a person evaluates their performance in front of others, usually in comparison to some over-valued benchmark. Due to errors in logic, people with low self-esteem focus on their own unfavorable characteristics, rather than focusing on their strengths. They also place a heavy value on what their friends think, and negative judgements from our friends can greatly influence the way we feel about ourselves. This emphasizes the importance of maintaining healthy peer groups, especially for children and teens.

*

So what if our job requires us to be good at dealing with people, as many jobs do, and we're really not very good at it? What if we just suck at dealing with people, like I have for most of my life? Fortunately, there's a solution. We can learn to be better at it. People who struggle with trying to figure out what to say to someone who is being difficult can improve their communication skills in this area. The best book that I've ever read on anxiety is *Anxiety Disorders and Phobias* by Dr. Aaron T. Beck, Dr. Gary Emery, and Dr. Ruth L. Greenberg. Dr. Aaron T. Beck is the father of cognitive therapy, and in his book he states that we have four basic choices of how to respond to others in a complex social interaction: to say nothing, to agree with them, to disagree, or to change the subject. It sounds like common sense, to know that we have these choices in dealing with other people, but I guess I never realized that I had a choice, and what I would have given to have known this twenty years ago.

The first choice is to say nothing, it's brilliant! I always felt that I had to respond in some way, but now I know how powerful silence can be. The next choice is simply to agree with the other person. This falls into the category of choosing your battles. If it doesn't really matter, just agree with them; "You know what, you're right, I'm an idiot, can we move on now?" Dr. Beck states that our next option, disagreeing with someone, is the most difficult one to take, because most people don't want to rock the boat. But you don't even have to defend your position if you don't want to, you can simply say, "Look, I just don't agree with you". Changing the subject is another interesting option which is also quite effective with children. I use this with my daughter when she's upset about something trivial like not getting a cookie - just change the subject and she forgets all about it.

I would also like to add a fifth choice which is one of my favorites that I use all the time, and that is responding with the statement, "I don't know". I always thought that admitting I didn't know something was a sign of weakness, and I would stress out about it and struggle to come up with the right answer. As amazing as I thought I was, I thought I should have all the answers. Now I give myself permission to admit ignorance, and it's a wonderful relief. This statement is also helpful if someone is trying to get you to make a decision on the spot. I always thought I had to give a definitive answer one way or the other, and I often would just say "yes", even though I didn't want to do something. Not letting yourself be forced to make a decision by saying, "I don't know, I'll think about it", is very empowering. But beware of abusing this one; saying "I don't know" too often could mean we're being lazy about making decisions and making commitments.

Besides learning how to use these basic communication tools, the key to overcoming social anxiety is to decrease the value we place on what others think of us, and increase the value we place on what we think of ourselves. At the end of the day, I try to remind myself of perhaps the best advice for people who suffer from social anxiety, in the words of Dr. Seuss, "Those who mind don't matter, and those who matter don't mind." When people judge or criticize me, I tell myself that I never really cared what those people thought about me before, so why should I care now? My true friends accept me with all my faults, and would never want to insult me or make me feel bad.

More Solutions

Nathaniel Branden once said, "Suffering in no achievement, joy is." We need to fix our problems, or let them go, and the best way to fix our problems and master our minds is by using cognitive behavioral therapy, or CBT. CBT is all about controlling our behavior by thinking better in response to anxiety. It's a lot like the Socratic Method which helps guide our thoughts down helpful pathways by asking the right questions, leading us to the right answers, resulting in more positive behaviors, and allowing us to realize that things aren't as bad as they seem. I often think of my anxiety as chaotic traffic congestion in my brain. The right questions will reroute the negative thoughts in a more positive direction and create roadways that lead to better flow, and thus better behavior. Another way to look at our anxious thoughts is to see them as children in our head having a fight, and they won't stop fighting until we sit everyone down, acknowledge and discuss what the problem is, and find an agreeable solution; this has to be done every time we feel anxious.

*

I've gotten to the point that I'm immediately aware of my anxiety. Now, I waste much less time trying to figure out if there's a problem that I need to fix; this way I can get back to feeling better again as soon as possible. It's important to understand that anxiety is the result of your brain telling you that it thinks something is wrong, and perhaps you should do something about it. But how exactly are you supposed to respond to these signals so that you can relieve your anxiety? Some advice says ignore your feelings or act as if you're not anxious, while others tell you that that's the worst thing to do, and that you should always acknowledge your feelings of anxiety. So what are you supposed to do? Well, both of these approaches are correct, it's just a matter of figuring out which situations require which approach. Initially, if you're anxious, the first step to overcoming it is always to acknowledge it to yourself. If you ignore anxious thoughts, then you usually end up feeling worse. Bad feelings are your brain's way of telling you something is wrong, so by admitting to yourself that you feel bad about something, you're sending a signal back to your brain that you got its message and that you will address the problem. This is the KEY! Once you tell your brain that you'll take care of the problem, you immediately start to feel better. Ignoring how you feel at this point will send a message to the brain that you're not going to fix the problem, then the brain has to send out a stronger signal, such as a bigger knot in your stomach, and you will feel worse without even realizing why. So acknowledging your anxiety and then patting yourself on the back for recognizing it is a good place to start.

Now that you've admitted to yourself that you're anxious and that there's a problem, the next key to feeling better is to figure out if there's anything you can do about it. If there's something you can do to fix the problem, then fix it; and if there's nothing you can do about it, you need to let it go. You have to send a message to your brain that, based on your review of the situation, there's nothing that you can do about it. By doing this, you're giving your brain permission to relax, and telling it that it doesn't have to worry about it anymore. If you're still anxious after you've told your brain there's nothing you can do about the problem, maybe you're missing something, so it's ok to clarify that there is, in fact, nothing you can do about it. If it's still bothering you after you've already gone over it, then you're probably obsessing about it, and here is where it's okay to ignore your anxious feelings so they go away.

Some people have trouble trusting themselves to let go of certain issues, and sometimes more than one message needs to be sent to the brain to tell it that you've examined the problem and determined that there's nothing you can do about it. I give myself two or three messages and then make myself forget about it by doing something that I enjoy. Sometimes I talk to myself like a good friend and say, "Look, we've already gone over this and there's nothing we can do, so just let it go for crying out loud." This took me forty years to figure out, so please don't underestimate it. Many people lose their minds because they spend most of their time worrying about things they can't do anything about. So if you want to keep it together, you have to let some things go. Oftentimes, the things we have trouble letting go of are things that have happened in the past, and these things can keep us from enjoying our present.

"Yesterday is history, tomorrow is a mystery, but today is a gift, that is why it is called the present" -Kung Fu Panda

We've all heard the helpful advice to live in the moment, or be in the "now". This sounds good, but it didn't help me until I understood exactly what *not* "living in the now" is, then I realized that it was how I've been living most my life, or perhaps I should say *not living it*. It sounds like common sense, but have you ever sat down and tried to figure out if this is how you're living your life? Is most of your time spent striving for some future goals that may or may not be met, and you will only truly be happy if you meet those goals, so you're struggling in the present to get to some place in the future that may not even exist? Don't get me wrong, goals are imperative to a high quality of life, but if your life is passing you by while you're somewhere else, then they're probably not worth it.

*

Don't lose sleep over your "dreams". Take it from someone who sees people die every day, if you're having nightmares about your "life's dreams", then they very well may be killing you. On the other hand, if you're having amazing dreams about your goals, and you can't wait to get out of bed in the morning to start creating your vision, then you're on the right track.

*

Another often helpful defense mechanism for overcoming anxiety is called dissociation, or separating yourself from a difficult situation by pretending as if you're watching your particular stressful situation unfold on TV. This allows you to think about it more rationally by making it less emotional. Be careful here though, because you don't ever want to be too disconnected from your reality.

*

Because working in an intensive care unit is so stressful and chaotic, one of my favorite tips, which I got from Richard Carlson in his book, *Don't Sweat the Small Stuff*, is to "practice being in the 'eye of the storm' ". I wonder if any of you have ever been in a hurricane, or seen actual film footage of the center of a hurricane passing over head, perhaps on some reality TV show of amazing survival stories. What happens right before the eye of the storm passes above you is complete and total chaos; it's a hurricane. But then, as the eye of the storm passes over you, it all stops; there's no wind, no rain, not even clouds. You can even see the stars as if it's the calmest night of the year. Then the hurricane comes back and everyone dies, but the point is that you can stay in the middle where it's calm, you just have to practice putting yourself there and bringing yourself back there when you stray, and you will stray because you're only human. I put a satellite picture of a hurricane in my studio to help me remember this.

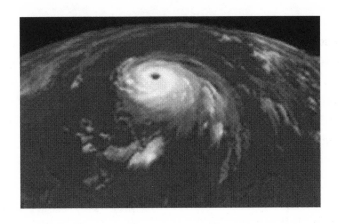

*

Another simple and effective thing you can do is breathe. We have all heard this advice before, but how often do we actually follow it? It's helpful to understand that we have a built-in reflex to hold our breath in response to an unpleasant stimulus. The cause for this is unknown, but I'm sure it goes back to the cavemen trying to avoid being seen by the cave bears. One of the first things I taught my daughter was to take a deep breath when she gets upset. Ironically, I often forget to do this myself. In the ICU, people have to do painful things all the time, like getting out of bed for the first time after having open heart surgery, and they always hold their breath. Holding your breath will always make the pain worse, whether it's from tubes in your chest or having a fight with your spouse, and breathing always makes things feel better. So when you catch yourself having a bad time, make it a point to breathe deeply. It's impossible to hold onto pain and negativity when you do this, which is precisely what you're doing when you hold your breath.

We must also learn how to handle problems *when* they occur. It's easy to know what to do when nothing's happening, the challenge is to do it in the heat of the moment. Shakespeare said it best, "All boats alike show mastership in sailing when the sea is calm".

If we can keep ourselves from ripping someone's head off when they piss us off, and instead handle the situation in a calm and Zen-like manner, we have to remember there will always be a chance that, the next time this happens, we may not handle the situation so well. Every now and then we're going to crack a little, but we can always reflect back on our more successful times and remind ourselves that even we are not perfect.

Complex problems are a little more stressful and challenging, and the best approach to dealing with them is to do what Joe Simpson did when he scratched and crawled his way back to base camp, he broke things down into small, concrete, manageable steps. Completion of each step allowed him to see that his goal could be reached as a result of his own effort and skill, increasing his confidence every step of the way. I always think of Joe when I'm struggling with something difficult and remind myself that almost nothing could be harder than what he went through. I keep telling myself, just make it to the next rock!!

Answer The *What Ifs*

So what if your dream position opened up at your company, but it requires public speaking, and you'd rather die than speak in public? You think to yourself, "If I take that position, I'll make a fool of myself, everyone will ridicule me, I'll be blackballed from my field, and I'll die cold and alone." Or what if this new girl you're dating, whom your head over heels for, has a best friend that's a guy, and he's gorgeous, funny, and amazing, and they can't stop laughing at each other while they're ignoring you every time you all are together? You think to yourself, "This girl is the one perfect person on Earth that I want to be with, and her best friend is so much more amazing than I am, why is she even dating me? I should just get in my car and drive off that cliff." I could go on forever with examples of complex and anxiety provoking situations that we all may find ourselves in. Those who aren't prepared to handle these situations will fail, as I did on countless occasions. Fortunately, one of the best teachers life can give us is failure, because the best experience for success is knowing what it's like to not succeed, and knowing that despite failing miserably, we dusted ourselves off and got back in the game.

There's no question that thinking positive is the best medicine, but this should also be combined with preparing for the worst, and there's no better way to prepare for failure than by answering the *what if* questions of life. Thinking well and controlling our consciousness will allow us to answer these questions with ease. When we ask ourselves, "What if this or that happens?", we must practice answering the questions in so much detail that it calms us to the point of never considering it again. There will be a few rare occasions when the answer to the question will be that we can't handle the outcome, then we can just do something different. But in most cases, the answer to the question will be far more tolerable than the dark and formless fear that's left in place of not answering the question in the first place. We can tell ourselves, "If I fail, this will happen, and then that will happen, and I will be able to handle it, and it will be worth it to give it a shot." All of this will give us the strength to get up on stage, fall flat on our face, stand back up, take a graceful bow, and keep on going. Sometimes, you might want to just throw yourself on the floor in the first place to get it over with.

The Agitators

It's one thing to try and prepare yourself for the worst, but it can be really annoying when someone else is trying to prepare you for the worst. I like to call these people the "agitators". They're the ones who are always trying to get me to react in a negative way. I just smile and nod and think, "They're trying to agitate me and I will not be agitated, not today!" Unfortunately, the agitator is oftentimes myself.

Trying to eliminate my toxic, negative thoughts is sometimes like trying to kick a heroin habit. I'll do really well for a while, and then BAM, I lose it. I'll be rolling along for weeks spewing sunshine on everyone, then out of the blue, everything sucks. Some people have to work a lot harder than others to control this, and that's just the way it is.

One of my favorite characters on Saturday Night Live is Debbie Downer, played by actress Rachel Dratch. If you're not familiar with her, she's the agitator. Her chronic negativity can ruin every happy and special moment that arises. At times, it felt like her character was based on me, and as I was watching the news religiously twice a day, and reading the paper cover to cover, I was well versed in every horribly tragic event that was occurring all over the world, and I wouldn't hesitate to tell you all about it in graphic detail. I was so good at my descriptions of tragedy that I could make you feel like you were really there and it actually happened to you.

One evening, I was out to dinner with some friends. I had spent the night before watching a fascinating television special on how diamonds were acquired in Sierra Leone, Africa. Some of the diamond companies obtained their supply of diamonds by having the poor local tribesman and their children dive underwater while breathing some ancient carbon monoxide apparatus, that would eventually kill them, to get the diamonds. At dinner that night, my friend Jim was talking about how he had just proposed to his girlfriend who was also there, and she was showing everyone her diamond engagement ring. Of course, the narcissist in me had to steal some of the attention and tell my horribly tragic blood diamond story that I had just learned about. After I was done telling the story, no one said anything and everyone looked like they wanted to throw up. I was just trying to share an interesting story, but I killed the special moment. Jim and his wife-to-be were more than a little insulted, and they never spoke to me again after that. Nice job Debbie. Not long after that, I was watching Saturday Night Live and a *Debbie Downer* skit came on. It was the one where she's at Thanksgiving dinner with her family and her brother pulls out a diamond engagement ring and proposes to his girlfriend. Debbie Downer's response was that they should all consider the lives lost in the African blood diamond trade, and the famous "wah, wah" sound played after her comment. Her negativity went on and on until everyone just left the table, leaving Debbie sitting there alone. I couldn't believe it; it was a caricature of myself. I really didn't want to be like that anymore, and it wasn't just my negative comments about current events, the negativity seeped into almost every one of my thoughts and comments; it was everywhere, all the time.

Now don't get me wrong, we all need to vent our frustrations from time to time, and misery really does love company, but bad company is bad company, and surrounding yourself with people who only agree with your negativity just breeds more negativity; this world has enough of that already. Being negative gives us some immediate gratification and satisfies our *id*, but this will be a net loss for our ego, and nothing of value will be gained unless it's followed up with something positive. The only thing life really gives us credit for is how hard we work at making ourselves and the people around us happy, and this is accomplished by problem solving, not agitating. So try to catch yourself the next time you're going to say something negative and ask yourself if you're going to accomplish anything worthwhile by saying it. If the answer is no, then can it.

Anger

"For every minute you're angry, you give up sixty seconds of peace of mind" -Ralph Waldo Emerson

My father was a man of few words. He didn't speak unless it was absolutely necessary, and when he did, you didn't get much. When we all sat down at the dinner table, there was silence, except for the sound of my father devouring his dinner; clearly he was trying to fill a deep void. Every time I catch myself inhaling my food I think of him... and I wonder if I'm doing the same thing. After weeks or months of barely speaking at all, my father would quietly go down into our unfinished basement, close the door, and launch into an explosion of rage. He would yell, scream, and swear at the vast, empty void of our basement. No one ever saw it coming, and you couldn't even understand what he was talking about, or who his anger was directed at, but it was the loudest yelling I've ever heard in my life. It would echo off the unfinished cement foundation, and the walls would shake. I would hide under my bed and pray it would end, which it did, after about a half hour. Then, my father would emerge from the gallows, looking still enraged but again silent, with eyes and veins popping out of his head. I can't remember exactly what he would do after that, but he would just disappear for a while, and no one ever talked about what happened.

So you won't be surprised when I tell you that I have a problem with controlling my anger and communicating with other human beings. But I don't want to blame it all on my father here, my mother was also a complete disaster with controlling her temper. Listening to my parents drift between talking to each other and having an argument was like listening to a poorly scripted made-for-TV movie. It would swing between cordial but apathetic small talk and some kind of horrible noises that raccoons make when they're fighting with each other. I sat by helplessly watching these episodes throughout my childhood, while an imprint of how I thought everyone should behave was being made on my brain. Needless to say, I've had a lot of work to do on myself.

Some people have a lower threshold for getting angry than others do. As with most human characteristics, part of it is inherited and the other part is learned from our environment, especially by the way we were raised by our parents. When we get really angry, it's often an accumulation of several different triggers, with each one sending out a wave of powerful chemicals into our bloodstream. Before the first wave has a chance to dissipate, the second one comes, and then the third one, with each one building upon the last, until an overwhelming "flood" of negative emotions and powerful natural chemicals overwhelms our rational brain, turning us into the Hulk.

From spending most of my time watching TV as a child, one of my favorite shows was *The Incredible Hulk*. I remember when Bill Bixby was trying to change a flat tire in the rain and he couldn't get the lug nuts off. When the crowbar slipped out of his hand, that was it, his eyes would turn scary monster blue and he would turn into the Hulk. I remember at the beginning of each episode, the word "ANGER" was the first thing you could see on the screen, and then the camera would pull out to show the whole word "DANGER" on the gamma ray device.

It didn't take too much to get Bill Bixby's character to crack, and while many of us have a low threshold for getting upset, others are almost impossible to rile up. But when our buttons are pushed, a flood of the neurotransmitters epinephrine and dopamine begin coursing through our veins and can turn us into a monster that can kill and destroy anything in its path. At this point, it's quite difficult for anyone to talk any sense into us.

An effective way to derail the rage process is to envision how ridiculous we would look turning into the Hulk, or a Paleolithic caveman, because part of this defense mechanism is tied to that time period when we understood that the best way to overcome our opponent was to kill them. These prehistoric responses are embedded in our DNA and unleash a storm of powerful chemicals that seem to give us the power to break a tree trunk in half. Unfortunately, this primal defense mechanism that saved our lives thirty thousand years ago is killing us now. It can throw a blood clot to our brain, or blow a hole in a blood vessel, then the Hulk will need to be spoon fed and have its diapers changed. Every time we get upset like this, at the very least, it takes years off our lives. Perhaps considering this fact may derail the rage train. It would also be helpful to envision ourselves as a prehistoric cave-child, because these overreactions are also very immature, often relating to our childhood when we didn't get our way and we threw a temper tantrum. The narcissistic "my way or the highway" mentality, and the lack of empathy that prevents us from seeing another's point of view, creates within us unrealistic expectations of others which triggers our rage.

Once the rage process starts and the chemicals are released within our body, it takes a little while for them to disappear after we've started the process of calming ourselves down. It's like doing a couple of lines of cocaine - the effect of the drug doesn't just stop at some point - it slowly wears off. Like trying to stop a freight train, the faster we're going and the more enraged we are, the longer it takes to stop the train.

In the United States, a woman is assaulted every nine seconds, and almost two people are murdered every hour of every day. Rage is responsible in many of these cases, so slowing things down and giving ourselves a timeout is imperative.

Fortunately, like any form of energy, rage can be transformed into something productive, rather than destructive. Lewis Presnall states in his book, *Search For Serenity*, "The explosive force in gasoline can blow up a building or it can be used to drive an automobile (...). In learning to control anger, it is necessary to harness the energy and slow the reaction of the explosion". But if we are unable to transform our anger into something more positive, then we have to just let it go. We can't hold onto it forever, and the sooner we let it go, the better. Buddha once said, "Holding onto anger is like grasping a hot coal with the intent of throwing it at someone else; you are the one who gets burned."

It's easy to think that merely having all this information will change your behavior and change your life, but having read just about every self-help book ever written, I can say from experience that's not true. I thought it would be, but reading all those books did little in terms of improving my sense of well-being. What I failed to realize is that I had to actually change the deeply ingrained pathways of negative thinking in my brain, tracks that were laid down twenty or thirty years ago, many in childhood, tracks that I've been riding over and over again. The process of change is quite slow and often difficult. Watch yourself then next time someone really pisses you off and see how you respond, despite already knowing how you should respond. I guarantee that you will be quite surprised at how difficult it is in the heat of the moment. I still have to practice smiling, speaking calmly, and saying something helpful to someone, when all I really want to do is rip their head off. But each time I do this, I'm changing my brain and increasing the probability that I will behave the same ideal way in the future.

When we're enraged we're also holding our breath, so taking a deep breath is a good place to start when we feel ourselves getting amped up. It's impossible to be angry and relaxed at the same time, and taking deep breaths relaxes us. Being grateful for what we have also makes it more difficult to get angry when things don't go our way. At the end of the day, we can't let our inability to control our emotions ruin our lives. We have to take responsibility for our own happiness; if we're angry because our life sucks, it's usually our own fault, and no one can fix it but us.

Taking Responsibility

To take responsibility for our own actions and behaviors means to be accountable for things that are within our control. It is impossible to be accountable while at the same time playing the role of victim, but many people spend a good portion of their lives blaming anything or anyone outside of themselves for their problems. This is very convenient because it doesn't require any action to be taken on the complainer's part. They can sit on the couch all day long and blame their spouse, their boss, their friends or the government, with the sole purpose being to perpetuate inactivity. The moment one takes responsibility for their life and happiness, is the moment that requires some sort of action on their part, either mental or physical, because they will either be letting something go and will now have free time on their hands with which to do something productive, or they will have to fix a problem that they themselves have created.

Nathaniel Branden discussed taking responsibility in his book, *Honoring The Self*. He described how taking responsibility involves considering the consequences of our actions, and that if everyone considered the consequences of their actions before they did something they would regret, they would never do it in the first place. Considering the consequences of our actions takes a little extra time. It requires slowing things down, especially in the heat of the moment. Our culture has placed a great emphasis on increasing the speed of just about everything. Faster cars, planes, trains, faster computers, and faster phones. We've come to value faster talking and thinking, and faster problem solving and decision making. We even teach our children to "think quick on their feet". The problem is that we've forgotten one of the fundamentals rules of life, and that is if you can't do something well slowly, then you can't do it well fast.

The idea of slowing things down goes back to Socrates and also has its roots in eastern philosophy, as well as in the martial arts such as Tai Chi, but it can be applied to most things in life. I used to ride a motorcycle and I remember when I got my first bike. My friend Billy, who was a Tai Chi instructor, told me that the best way to practice riding my bike was to go as slow as I could around an obstacle course without putting my feet down and losing my balance. If I perfected this, he said, only then would I be able to go faster safely. So we have to do the opposite of what our brains have been trained to, which is to respond as quickly as possible, and slow down our reaction times. If we pretend we are watching ourselves on TV, in the heat of the moment, we have to hit the *slow-motion* button so that we have time to see and process the potential consequences of our actions. Then we can avoid doing or saying something we'll surely regret. Since I've started doing this myself, it's been fascinating watching how some people act when they're getting amped up over a conversation they're having with me. Slowing things down keeps me calm and often throws the other person off because they're expecting me to get amped up with them.

By considering the consequences of our actions, we'll make fewer mistakes and blunders, and when we do screw up, we'll be much more likely to own up to it. Best of all, by taking more time to think things through, we'll be changing our brain for the better.

Change Your Mind, Change Your Brain

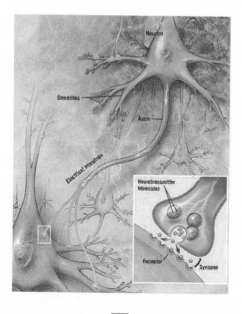

Until now, the scientific community believed that changing the brain was impossible. But recent breakthroughs in brain research indicate that, without a doubt, one can change their brain, even after severe neurological damage. This process is called brain plasticity.

When we're mastering our minds, we're in essence training ourselves to be our own psychotherapist, and while we're having these conversations with ourselves in our head, we're actually changing the structure inside our brain. Not that there's anything wrong with actually talking to a therapist, but what they will do is teach us how to be our own therapist, and that's what mastering our mind is all about.

There is nothing more inspiring to me than knowing that when I accomplish a difficult task, when I give up a bad habit, and when I teach myself to control my thinking, my brain scan will be different afterwards, and there will be visible changes from the new pathways that have been formed, as well as the bad ones that have been erased.

Being miserable has a lot to do with something that Norman Doidge discusses in the best book ever written on brain plasticity, *The Brain That Changes Itself,* and that is how our thoughts often go down the same old negative pathways, leading to bad habits, and causing us to feel like crap. Dr. Doidge explains that once our thoughts go down a pathway, it becomes easier for our brain to choose this pathway that has already been created, whether good or bad. So it's up to us to prevent the creation and use of bad pathways, and instead make new pathways that lead to positive thinking and good habits. For example, if you're trying to kick a bad habit, the trick is to make a substitution with something that is equally or more enjoyable as the bad habit, thus filling the void left behind from removing the bad habit. Instead of smoking a cigarette first thing in morning, put your favorite song on and do something else with your hands that you love to do and don't spend enough time doing, like playing the guitar or building something. Think of how hard it is to be productive with a cigarette in your hands. It's hard for most people, except my mother, to play with their child or their dog or their guitar with a cigarette in their hands. Of course, this also requires having a well-developed list of things that you love to do that are healthy as well; it requires having a hobby that requires both hands so one is not free to hold a cigarette.

It's also helpful to undervalue whatever it is that you're getting out of the bad habit, and crank up the volume on the benefits you're getting out of the good habit. Remind yourself of the trillion or so free radicals that each puff of a cigarette delivers to your lungs and brain, or how inconvenient it is to take the elevator downstairs and go outside when the temperature is 20 degrees to smoke a cigarette at work. If you have a bad habit of constantly arguing with your spouse, you can remind yourself that having a temper tantrum provides a little immediate gratification, but the damage it incurs to the relationship could take years to repair, and handling the disagreement appropriately is very rewarding and challenging, and quite impressive as well. It's also helpful to remember that having a temper tantrum is super easy, which is why three-year-olds do it all the time. At the end of the day though, it's not always easy to avoid going down pathways that have been there for twenty, thirty, or forty years; but it's not impossible either.

If you think changing your brain to break a bad habit is hard, imagine how difficult it is for someone who had a stroke and cannot move the entire left side of their body. They have to rebuild pathways that have been completely destroyed. If they can do it, you can too, so it's time to stop making excuses and get to work.

Fear

Now, how about another piece of misery pie? At the bottom of the pie, underneath the layers of anger and anxiety, lies fear. Part of taking responsibility for ourselves and our lives means facing and overcoming our fears. From Little Miss Muffet's fear of spiders, to our social fears of speaking in public, many fears are not nearly as scary as we think they are. By shining the light of our consciousness on our fears, we will be able to see them for what they are, something much less ominous than what they seemed to be in the dark. Wrestling with fears as an adult is hard enough, but being a parent and trying to allay our child's fear can be even more challenging, so the better we are at conquering our own fears, the better we will be at teaching our child to conquer theirs.

My mother was a worry wort, and everything seemed impossible and scary to her, so I learned at a young age that I had no control over my life, and that most things should be feared. Fortunately, I learned that as long as fear is undefined, it retains its power. So exposing our fears for what they are will take away their power. When we ask ourselves, "What am I afraid of?" the actual process of identifying and defining the fear destroys it, causing it to collapse into something tangible, something we can contain and manage, rather than the shapeless blob of slaughter it was before.

"Nothing in life is to be feared, it is only to be understood. Now is the time to understand more, so that we may fear less." - Marie Curie

A miserable existence is peppered with fear. Some fears are bigger than others, like being afraid that your abusive partner is going to kill you, since this happens to thousands of women every year in the U.S. alone. You could be afraid that you're going to be sexually assaulted, since this happens to almost one in four women at some point in their lives. You could simply have a generalized fear of dying in any of a number of horribly tragic ways, since we are constantly bombarded with these stories on the news. Our power lies in reminding ourselves that, of course, there's always a small chance something bad can happen to us, but there are also many things that we can do prevent those things from happening. If we're in an abusive relationship, then we can stick up for ourselves and refuse to be abused. We can start making plans to leave and figure out how to take care of ourselves and our children with help from the community. If we're afraid of being assaulted, we can take a self-defense class and buy a stun gun. The point is that we can *do* something about it. Taking action will give us the confidence to know that we can handle whatever life throws at us. But we can't spend every moment of our lives trying to fix our fears. We have to remind ourselves that there's only so much we can do to keep ourselves safe. At some point, our efforts will have to be good enough so that we can finally move on with our lives.

Facing the fear of being physically assaulted is at the far end of the extreme, but many people's lives are ruled by fears of just about anything, or even nothing at all. I spent a good portion of my life being afraid of just about everything from the moment I woke up in the morning. I created a life of chronic distractions from my fears. Bad relationships and a lot of bad TV filled the core of most of my days, all while life was quietly passing me by; I should have feared that the most. No one that I associated with was going to tell me that something was wrong with me because they were all screwed up themselves. So after half a lifetime of waking up with a knot in my stomach, I finally realized that I wasn't going to magically start feeling better. I had to put facing my fears at the top my list; I was determined to become an expert at it. The turning point came when I went back to school. School was a perfect distraction from my anxiety, but it was also something that I was good at, and most importantly, it was there that I learned about the anatomy of fear.

Chapter 9

AMYGDALA

Despite how horribly unpleasant the experience of fear is, it's ironic how many people go out of their way to feel it. Last Halloween, we visited one of our local amusement parks and I was shocked to learn about a terrifying virtual-reality attraction that we had just missed. It had you strapped down in a wheelchair to virtually live through being involuntarily committed to an insane asylum, with bloody bodies lying all over the floor, insane people moaning in pain, and crazy people running all over the place. God knows what else happened inside those virtual-reality goggles, but the "attraction" was removed due to public outcry from the mental health community who complained that the park was turning mental illness into a horror show. Surprisingly, thousands of people unsuccessfully petitioned to keep the attraction open because they thought it was so great.

I wonder if those *fear seekers* realized what that fear was doing inside their bodies. According to a study published in the British Medical Journal, watching horror movies is associated with an increase of blood coagulant factor VIII. Our bodies increase this clotting factor when we're scared to prevent us from bleeding to death in the event that what we're afraid of is going to tear us limb from limb. This worked out well for us when we were fending off the cave bears, but the problem now is that we're not usually going to bleed to death from whatever it is we're afraid of. So every time we feel fear, our chance of getting a blood clot increases, and getting a blood clot is one of the most frequent causes of death for us modern humans. Think about that the next time you take your children to a scary movie. But even if we don't go out of our way to feel fear, imagine what the effects of a lower level of fear can do to us over the course of a lifetime. This makes it even more important for us to understand fear so that we can get a handle on it.

The part of the brain that is most responsible for our unpleasant feelings, emotions, and behaviors is the amygdala. The amygdala, or amygdalae (pleural because there's one on each side of your brain), are almond shaped (amygdala means almond in Latin) groups of cells located deep within the temporal lobes of the brain in humans. Even though there are two of them, I will be referring to them in the singular *amygdala*, just because it sounds better. The amygdala plays an important part in creating memories and having emotional reactions. The role it plays in memory is by facilitating increased retention of an event when it is associated with greater emotional arousal. This is one of the reasons scary things are so hard to forget. BOO!! See, now you'll never forget this.

The amygdala is different in men vs. women. Men have a greater number of connections to their right amygdala and women have a greater number of connections to their left amygdala. The right amygdala is associated with greater visual/spatial related input, as well as greater physical responses to emotional stimuli. This may be illustrated by the fact that men react more aggressively to stress. The left amygdala is associated with greater language abilities, which could be why women tend to want to talk things out more than men do. But whether you're a man or a woman, the amygdala seems to play a critical role in many psychological disorders, such as social anxiety, obsessive compulsive disorders, and post-traumatic stress. Simply put, the amygdala is most famous for eliciting the emotion of fear. In fact, people with damage to their amygdala, such as people with the rare Urbach-Weithe disease, may go through their entire lives without ever experiencing fear. These people would walk straight through the flames of a burning building to save someone without a second thought, which sounds really heroic, the only problem is that they'll die in the process. The fear is there for a reason, and without it we'd all be recklessly putting our lives in danger.

Fear becomes a problem when the chaos in our minds gets out of control and we overreact to certain emotional triggers, this is when the amygdala "emotionally hijacks" the rational part of our brain - an idea discussed by Daniel Goleman in his book, *Emotional Intelligence*. When we get a strong stimulus, it is first sent to the amygdala or the emotional brain, initially bypassing the rational part of our brain - the prefrontal cortex. The reason it is sent to the amygdala first is a survival mechanism so that we can react quickly to a threat without spending too much time thinking about it. The problem is that the amygdala, if left unchecked, can be far more powerful than the rational brain.

Research has found that some animals' amygdala can respond to a stimulus in as quick as twelve thousandths of a second, far faster than the prefrontal lobe can operate. This is great if a sabretooth tiger is about to jump on us and we react with, "If I kill it, it won't kill me", or if a deer jumps out in front of our car when we're driving. But this often gets us into trouble in our regular daily lives because our interpretation of the stimulus is often distorted, and it is distorted because we haven't taken enough time to rationally think about it.

If the amygdala recognizes the stimulus as something threatening, then the amygdala triggers a flood of hormones and "hijacks" the rational brain, or the prefrontal cortex. One of the hormones that is triggered by the amygdala is adrenaline, or epinephrine, a substance so powerful that it's the main drug we use in the ICU to bring someone back to life after their heart stops beating, so imagine what it can do to you in the middle of an emotional hijack.

Let's say you're a really insecure guy and you're out at a bar with your girlfriend and some guy hits on her; the "kill" instinct can immediately be triggered. This response by the amygdala occurs within milliseconds and much sooner than the rational brain has a chance to intervene. So if a stimulus is perceived as a threat, i.e. the guy's telling really funny jokes and you suck at telling jokes and your girlfriend thinks he's hysterical, the amygdala reacts before any possible direction from the rational brain can be received, and the "kill the guy" message is sent to your body and a bar brawl ensues. If, however, the amygdala does not consider the stimulus a threat - perhaps because the guy hitting on your girlfriend isn't very funny and has a mustache, and you know your girlfriend hates mustaches - then the amygdala acts according to the directions received from the rational part of the brain, and you tell yourself, "Calm down, there's no need to kill the guy". Or what if you have to give a speech to an audience for the first time ever and you're terrified of public speaking? You step up on stage and look at all those people staring at you. Fear strikes via the amygdala and you think, "Oh crap, I'm gonna bomb this and my career will be ruined!" Your heart starts racing, you're breathing too fast, and you pass out. Your career is now over, and you will be on disability for the rest of your life. Keeping the amygdala in check is crucial to mastering our minds, so to get a better idea of how to do this, let's take a look at how the military handles it.

Think Like a Navy Seal

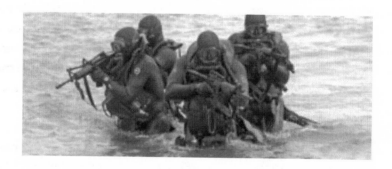

Few would argue that one of the best ways to stimulate your amygdala is to have someone try to kill you, and there's no better place to experience that than in combat warfare. But if there are no battles going on, then going through Navy Seal training would get you as close to the real thing as possible. Fortunately, most of us won't have to experience this degree of stress in our lifetimes, although sometimes it feels like it, and many everyday situations can mimic this type of stress. Not that anything compares to trying to survive in combat as a Navy Seal, but trying to make it home during rush hour on Friday afternoon on the Kennedy Expressway in downtown Chicago, or being a critical care nurse, or even arguing with our spouse are a few examples of amygdala triggering events for us mere mortals. So I think that learning how the elite special forces handle having someone trying to kill them is the best place to learn how to handle life.

When a stressful event triggers the amygdala, an enormous dose of adrenaline is injected into our veins, our blood pressure sky rockets, and our heart starts pounding out of our chest. You can see the force of the heart beating, you can feel it, and you can hear it. In fact, if the heart beats fast enough and strong enough, in extremely rare cases and in people who already have weak hearts, it can explode in what's called spontaneous left ventricular rupture. If your heart doesn't explode, it can sometimes simply start to fail from continuously high doses of adrenaline in response to an overwhelmingly stressful situation, such as the loss of a loved one. This has come to be known as "broken heart syndrome" in the medical community, or Takotsubo Cardiomyopathy. These cases are extremely rare, but they do happen, and I'll never forget the few young people that I've taken care of, whose hearts were failing for no apparent reason, other than the loss of a loved one, or simply the stress of their lives. Most of us, however, will handle very stressful situations every now and then just fine, with no damage to our heart, but many smaller stresses, happening continuously over a lifetime can wreak havoc in our bodies if we handle them poorly. So how can we learn to have more control over this power of the mind?

Being an expert catastrophizer myself, I love to consider worst case scenarios because if I can handle that, I can handle anything. So consider the most horrible situation of your choice, whether it's trying to escape from Auschwitz, North Korea, or Afghanistan, the more dysfunctional and negative your thinking is, the faster your heart will be beating, and the more adrenaline will be pumped into your veins. If you can't handle it, then past a certain point, you will lose control of everything, and this is what Navy Seals have to overcome.

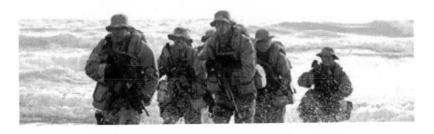

One of the most fascinating documentaries that I've ever seen is called *The Brain* featured on the History Channel. It describes how the Navy Seals were having trouble getting their prospective candidates to pass the hardest part of the program, and many of them were giving up and dropping out because they couldn't handle the stress. What they had to do for their final exam was to dive into a pool with their face masks and oxygen tanks on, while the enemy (their instructor) harassed them under the water by hitting them and pushing them around, getting their heart rates up by continuously bullying them. Then the enemy would rip the trainees' masks off and tie their oxygen hoses in a knot so there wasn't enough length in the hose to put their oxygen masks back on. At this point, they couldn't take another breath until they somehow got their masks untangled and back on their face. So to pass the test, the trainees had to remain calm, talk themselves through untying the knot, and put their masks back on, all the while knowing that if they couldn't do it, they would die, and they had to do it while still being physically harassed by their instructors. I'm not sure if there's anything more stressful than not being able to breathe, and many soldiers failed the test.

In the Intensive Care Unit, we deal with people all the time that are having trouble breathing. These people get what has come to be known in the medical field as a "sense of impending doom"; they're convinced they're going to die, and this is what happened to the soldiers. Their amygdala took over, pushing their heart rates up off the charts, using up all their oxygen, and they freaked out, as of course anyone under these circumstances would. But they weren't just anyone, they were Navy Seals, and they had to figure out how to overcome their fears. So what the Navy Seals did was hire a psychologist to teach the instructors how to get the soldiers to have more control over their own minds.

Not surprisingly, what the Navy Seals learned was that most of their problems were directly linked to the amygdala. What was happening to the trainees was that their amygdala was being hijacked by the fear response, jacking up their heart rates way too high, and creating chaos in their minds so that their rational mind became useless. The instructors had to learn how to teach the trainees to override their amygdala so that their rational mind could stay in control, and the part of the brain that is capable of overriding the amygdala is the frontal lobe – this is where the rational brain resides. The frontal lobe is responsible for things such as task performance, planning, motivation and reasoning. They needed to get the frontal lobe working better, and in order to do this, they focused on four main areas of training.

The first was goal setting – this is where frontal lobe reasoning brings structure to chaos, keeping the amygdala in check. They had to get that mask back on no matter what, without letting anything stop them. The next step was mental rehearsal. By reviewing in their minds exactly what they needed to do to get their mask back on, by visualizing the entire experience, they were actually doing two things. First, they were desensitizing themselves to the unpleasant aspects of the experience. Second, by visualizing exactly what they had to do to reach their goal, it was like they were actually doing it, over and over again. So when the time came to really do it, it was like they were old pros. Being harassed by their instructors had to be no big deal to them, like shooing flies away; that's the desensitization working. Then, they had to calmly hold their breath long enough to untangle their oxygen hoses so they could put their masks back on. Being calm uses much less oxygen, and when you only have one breath's worth, there isn't any to lose on freaking out. Finally, they had to systematically untangle the oxygen hose, step by step, as they had already done a million times in their minds, and put their masks back on.

The third aspect of the training was aimed at self-talk, that is how the trainees talked to themselves in their heads during the task. Positive "can do" thoughts can override the negative fearful signals from the amygdala. This may sound like it would be easy to do, but when someone is trying to kill you, it's not. So instead of thinking, "Holy Shit! I'm going to die because I'll never be able to do this", they say to themselves, "You can do this, you're totally prepared and YOU CAN DO IT!"

The last part of the training focuses on physical arousal control. When we're stressed, the amygdala tries to jack up our blood pressure and heart rate and get us to breathe fast and shallow. Breathing fast and shallow increases the blood flow to the amygdala and feeds its fury. By deliberately breathing slowly and deeply, we're slowing down our heart rates and counteracting the amygdala. Obviously, the trainees couldn't use this trick because they were holding their breath, but otherwise, it's extremely useful. Slow deep breaths with long, slow exhales induce the relaxation response and increase blood flow to the part of the brain that needs it the most, the prefrontal lobe - the rational brain. Brain scans have shown that when the amygdala is triggered, more blood flows to it than to the prefrontal cortex. We want to reverse this and get as much flow to the rational brain as possible. So if you take nothing else away from this discussion, at the very least... take a deep breath.

The Silver Lining

The amygdala has been getting a bad rap lately, but even though we're not cavemen anymore, we still need it to keep us out of danger. We can't just have it removed or we would all be fearless and reckless, jumping off cliffs, driving like maniacs, and walking through fires. So we need to learn how to live with the amygdala. We need to appreciate its power, but we don't always have to take its bate. We also need to appreciate the evolutionary speed with which the amygdala sends us messages. This speed will always be faster than the speed that our prefrontal cortex sends us rational messages. Fortunately, while our prefrontal cortex may not be faster than the amygdala, it's much smarter than the amygdala. Using Freud's analogy of how the ego controls the id like a man controls the great power of a horse, our prefrontal cortex can rein in the power of the amygdala, thus channeling its energy more productively.

*

Another way of understanding how we can get a handle on the amygdala is by understanding the process of reappraisal. Reappraisal involves first becoming aware of the amygdala's knee jerk thoughts of doom and gloom. Going back to our Navy Seal recruits for example, when their oxygen masks are ripped off, the amygdala sends them the message, "YOUR GONNA DIE!" By first becoming aware of this overreaction and saying to ourselves, "Okay, you're freaking out dude; it's not that bad; let's chill and do what we've been trained to do because we can handle this." This is a reappraisal of the situation and sets the stage for a more favorable outcome.

Reappraisal is an indispensable tool that can be used when we're alone and struggling with our thoughts internally, or when we're having a difficult interaction with someone else. Our emotional reaction to an event is determined by our interpretation of the meaning and significance of the event. So if we feel like crap about something, it's because we're negatively appraising the situation. Some people are lucky and their general appraisals tend to be positive most of the time. Many people though, like myself, have to always struggle to see the silver lining. People who have negative initial appraisals can improve their ability to positively reappraise a situation. This is helpful with the many irritating things that happen to us in the course of a day. If someone cuts you off while you're driving, after getting pissed off and before you flip them off, you could consider that perhaps they're on their way to the hospital to see a sick loved one. If someone says something rude to you, before you tell them to screw off, you could consider that perhaps you misunderstood them. Reappraisal is intertwined with slowing things down and considering the consequences of our actions. This process exposes opportunities that exist, which may only last fractions of a second, for a positive reappraisal to avert certain disaster, or to prevent a hurtful comment from coming out of our mouths that could start a nuclear war and change the course of our lives forever.

The difference between cool, calm, and collective people and "hot heads" is their ability to break these events down to their atomic structure by pressing the slow-motion button in their minds so that they can get a better view of what's really happening. These people are able to take control of the moment before it gets out of hand. Practice and discipline will help us increase our awareness of when we are being triggered so that we can respond more favorably.

Every time our buttons are pushed must be seen as an opportunity to practice this, and the more we view these moments as part of a game, the more enjoyable the process will be. The bottom line is that our behavior is a matter of choice and responsibility. Regardless of what happens to us or what someone says to us, if we do or say something destructive, we're choosing to be an ass, and we must take responsibility for that.

Reappraisal is the key to feeling good about something when others would just feel bad. I like to call it the "slapping lipstick on a pig" trick of the mind to make things seem just a little bit better than they would otherwise. But it's not just about making ourselves feel better, it's about having more control of what's happening around us. Our ability to do this while we're calmly sitting back and pondering our lives is very important, but being able to master this ability during a stressful situation or in stressful encounters with others is priceless. In the end, it could very well add years to our lives.

Chapter 10

THE LAST DAY

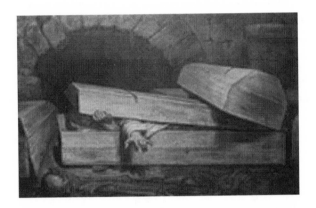

Someone once said that if you're going to live every day like it was your last, you should ask yourself the following question, "How do you know it isn't?" Like the cavemen surely were, we must be ever so aware of how fragile, uncertain, and short life is. The purpose is not to create fear and anxiety in our hearts, but to help put everything in its proper perspective, especially during those moments when we are angry, fearful, or anxious. So with that in consideration, here are a few more valuable insights that will help make one of our last days... one of our best days.

- Be patient. Opportunities to practice being patient happen all the time. Waiting around for an appointment or a date, or listening to your four-year-old tell you a really long story when you're running late, are excellent opportunities to break your habit of feeling impatient. Perhaps taking a few extra moments to listen to your daughter's story will actually be preventing you from getting into a car accident on your way to your very important appointment.

- Be thankful - "When you appreciate the good, the good appreciates" - Tal Ben-Shahar

- If you're fighting with your spouse, it's helpful to make yourself think about how much you love them (assuming you do). It's very difficult to hold love and anger in your heart at the same time.

- Don't waste time. Seeing people die every day at the hospital is like getting run over by a truck every day. It's devastating. It's soul-crushing. But it has also been ironically inspiring in that it has made me more aware than ever of how precious and short life really is. As a result, I have developed an extreme intolerance of wasted time. I often put pressure on myself if I think I'm doing something unnecessarily, or when I could be doing something more important. I'm also quite judgmental of others who seem to be wasting their time. Maybe this is wrong, and maybe if I heard these people acknowledge that they know they could die at any moment and they still choose to sleep all day, or sit on the couch and watch TV, that would be more acceptable. Some of these people have even had brushes with death and have been given a second lease on life, yet they still let time slip through their hands as if it was endless. Sometimes people put important things off for a "better" time, sometime next year or so, but it's important to know which things just aren't worth putting off because we might not be here then.

Worrying about stuff that doesn't really matter is also wasted time. If I'm worried about something, I often ask myself if it's something I'll give a crap about on my deathbed; the answer is usually "no", but if the answer is "yes" then I need to fix the problem so I don't regret it later on.

In the hospital, when we're not desperately trying to keep some people alive, we get a break from that by helping others die peacefully and naturally. It's a fascinating thing, standing by and quietly watching someone take their last few breaths. Every time I have the same thoughts... I wonder if everything worked out okay for them or if they had any regrets, then I wonder if everything will work out okay for me.

The strange thing is that, right after people die, they're dead. That's it; it's over and there's no turning back. During my nursing training, we were required to spend a day at the Coroner's Office to learn what their job is like. I have to say that this was one day that will forever be emblazoned on my brain, and I think everyone should have this experience, especially troubled youths. During our visit, we saw the complete autopsies of three people that were alive earlier that morning. One was the charred remains of someone who was killed in a car accident, probably by someone who was driving too fast and texting someone. The other was a 7-year-old boy who, just hours before, was alive and well and innocently riding his bicycle when he was hit by a car by someone who again, was probably driving too fast and on their cellphone. The last body was the victim of a gang shooting.

Before we saw the autopsies, the families were allowed to view the bodies. We were taken into a special room where we were able to watch the family of the gang shooting victim see their dead son and brother for the first time since they had died. I couldn't imagine how hard it was for them to see their loved one lying there on the cold hard slab of concrete, and I can still hear the echoes of their howling sobs. But as powerful as their tragic sorrow was, it could not turn back the hands of time and erase the unfortunate paths they all took to be there that day.

That day was the last day for a lot of people. I wondered what the guy who got shot thought about when he woke up that morning. Did he have a knot in his stomach? Did he say something mean and insensitive to his girlfriend, the one person who really loved him, and now he'll never have a chance to take it back? Was there anything else his mother wished she had said or done before he passed? I guess we'll never know. A trip to the coroner's office should be required for everyone.

Nothing can describe what it's like seeing dead people who were alive just a few hours or even a few minutes ago. Their transition happened so recently that you can almost feel this urge to reach back in time and help them avoid their ultimate fate, but you can't. It feels like you can because they just died and it's so close to the present, but it's in the past and you can't - it's too late. Then all you can do is just sit there in disbelief that such a brief moment in time can make the difference between life and death. So if that little voice inside your head tells you that if you don't do something you'll regret it, you better listen; and if it's the second time you've heard that little voice telling you the same thing because the first time you ignored it, you really should listen now.

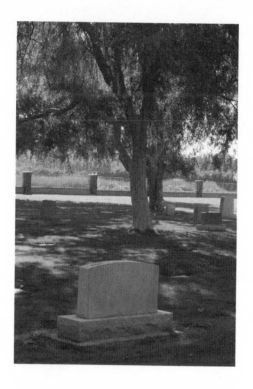

Chapter 11

RELATIONSHIP/COMMUNICATION

If you're still alive and planning on living a long time, it would be nice to spend that time with another person. Not that there's anything wrong with being single and living alone, but ultimately, it's nice to have someone else around. We get a dose of oxytocin and other cool brain chemicals that make us feel good when we're close to other people who know us well. But if you can't think well and don't talk pretty, it will be hard to sustain a healthy relationship with another human being.

Along with thinking well and controlling our emotions, learning how to communicate and deal with others doesn't usually make it very high on the list of learning priorities for schools. It has been taken for granted that we all somehow have an innate ability to talk, communicate, and respond to others properly. But the sad truth is that most of us suck at it. All the while we think we are master negotiators, and it's everyone else who is retarded.

I can only imagine the difference it would have made in my life if I knew how to talk and communicate well early on. Speaking well is an art, and talking to someone who has mastered it is rare and inspiring, and quite appealing as well. Every time we open our mouths to speak to another human being should be appreciated and respected for what it is: a precious opportunity to enhance that relationship; and we must be ever so aware that choosing the wrong words can have disastrous effects that can last a lifetime, especially when speaking to our children, which I will address in the parenting section. Right now, I want to focus on our primary relationship with our significant other, but keep in mind that everything is applicable to everyone we talk to.

Our relationship with the person we've chosen to spend our life with is crucial to our well-being and quality of life. If there's a problem here, it will cast a shadow on all other aspects of our life, so it must be rectified if we are to attain the greatest level of happiness.

Psychological Visibility

The cornerstone of any healthy relationship is psychological visibility, a term that most people have never heard of. I first learned about this from Nathaniel Branden, a psychotherapist who started the Branden Institute for Self-Esteem in Los Angeles. Dr. Branden sadly passed away while I was writing this book, but his spirit will be alive in me for the rest of my life, as it will be alive in the thousands of other lives that he touched. Dr. Branden was a pioneer of work on self-esteem and wrote over twenty books on relationships and self-esteem. He described psychological visibility as being able to see ourselves in others, and helping others see themselves in us. It is responsible for one of the best feelings one can get from another human being. It's like getting into a state of flow, but instead of working on a project, you're interacting with another human being. I also learned that the absence of psychological visibility was the reason I don't like talking to certain people because they make me feel invisible, like when they're talking to me I could just walk away and they wouldn't even notice I was gone, or when I start talking to them they ignore me or start talking to someone else. In fact, I realized that the absence of psychological visibility was responsible for every failed relationship that I've ever had.

So what is it exactly? Psychological visibility is the process of seeing ourselves, our values, the things we think are important, reflected back to us from another person who holds the same values. If we make a joke, and someone else laughs, we feel visible; we feel seen. If we're not in total denial about our appearance, most of us take pleasure in seeing our own reflection in the mirror, even if we don't like everything we see; it's a familiar face and we take comfort in that. In contrast, if we make a joke that we think is really funny, and no one laughs, we feel invisible, which is one of the most painful feelings we can experience psychologically. It goes back to when we were children and were ignored or misunderstood by our parents. We know when someone's not listening to us because we can feel it, and it hurts.

If you've ever read *The Little Prince* by Antoine de Saint Exupery, one of the best-selling books ever written, it starts out with an excellent example of feeling psychologically invisible. In the beginning of the book, at six years old and after reading a book about the jungle, the Little Prince draws a picture of boa constrictor that swallowed an elephant and he calls it his masterpiece. He shows his masterpiece to the "grown-ups" but the "grown-ups" assume it's a plain old hat, and encourage him to lay aside his drawings and instead devote himself to more important schoolwork. That's why, the Little Prince says, "at the age of six, I gave up what might have been a magnificent career as a painter."

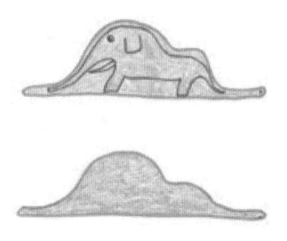

Making someone feel visible is one of the greatest gifts you can give another human being, especially children, but an intimate relationship cannot exist without it. So many people spend their entire lives feeling invisible to their partners, and then try to dull the pain in various destructive ways, such as over-eating, over-drinking, or over-medicating. If someone you're considering as a life partner doesn't laugh at your jokes, that's a red flag. If they don't care about the things you care about, then you have a problem, a big problem. If you're upset and in pain and your partner is oblivious to it after you have clearly told them you have a problem, and all you get is false reassurance like, "Don't worry, you'll feel better, it will all work out." Really? How? By me working my way out the door?

From learning about visibility, I've gained an amazing awareness of when people *get* me, and when they don't; of when someone is listening to me, and when they're just blankly staring at me while they're thinking about what they're going to say next. It's amazing how many times I try to tell someone a story, and before I can even finish, they start telling me a *better* story. Whatever your story is about, some people think they have a much more interesting one. One-upping people makes them feel invisible.

When people *get* us, when they really listen and respond appropriately, it can give us goose bumps. On the other hand, when we're trying hard to explain something important to someone, and despite our best efforts, they have no idea what we're talking about and their response has nothing to do with what we're talking about, it can be very disturbing and make us feel like we're alone on a deserted island.

Empathy

The key ingredient of psychological visibility is empathy. The degree of empathy that many people have is shockingly low. It can even be considered a global epidemic with the number of atrocities that seem to keep multiplying as the years go by. Maybe it's because of our desensitization by the media with one traumatic event after another, or the slaughterous video games that everyone seems to be playing. Like a crack addiction, we need stronger and stronger stimuli to have even a small empathetic response. It used to be that if you sprained your ankle people would throw you a "Get Well" party. Now you need to have your leg ripped off in a tractor accident to get a card in the mail. Fortunately, empathy is making its way back to the top of the list of essential qualities that successful people must possess. It's hard to run a successful business if you can't make your clients feel understood.

Perhaps most important is that the depth of our close relationships will be wafer thin without it.

Part of the problem is that many people don't even know what *empathy* means. It is often confused with *sympathy* or feeling sorry for someone, but that's not it. Empathy is the insightful awareness of another person's thoughts and feelings, and the ability to convey that understanding to the other person. It's letting them know that *you know how they feel*, not by "one-upping" their story with one of your own, but by saying to them, "Wow, you must really feel awful after what happened; it must be hard to be going through what you're going through." It's the ability to make someone who's in pain feel a little bit better because they know you understand how they feel. Last but not least, it's the ability to suppress the urge to "fix" someone's problems yourself, and instead get them to talk about how they feel. When people talk about how they feel, solutions often reveal themselves, and you will be helping them fix their own problems, which is much more rewarding for them. The bottom line is that tuning yourself in to how other people feel is the easiest way to improve your relationship with everyone.

Forgiveness

"Forgiveness is the fragrance a violet sheds on the heel that has crushed it" -Mark Twain

Forgiveness is another ingredient that the recipe of a good relationship cannot do without. Of course, if someone has maliciously hurt or insulted you, that's another story, but as a general rule, no one is perfect and we all from time to time say and do really stupid things. I guarantee that you and your partner or your friend are going to piss each other off. I can also guarantee you that if forgiveness is not part of the equation, the relationship will fall apart. You have to cut each other some slack.

To Talk or Not To Talk?

One of the biggest roadblocks to communication is spending too much time talking about our opinions, and spending too little time making the other person feel heard. This is another vital facet of psychological visibility and empathy. Until this takes place, until we make the other person feel *understood*, it doesn't matter how much we say because we will be wasting our breath. I've spent most of my life sucking at this, and I still have to continuously remind myself that I should listen and clarify better. Because I think I'm so smart and have so much intelligent information to share, I always thought that people would be so amazed that I'm speaking to them in the first place that they would automatically take what I said and spread it to the rest of the world. I always used to complain about how "no one listens to me", then I realized that *I* was the problem. I still have to fight my own sense of entitlement by insisting that I should be understood first. The sooner I give this up, the sooner I will be understood.

Listen to me when I tell you that it's hard listening to other people when you're so focused on yourself. The next time you're talking to someone, try asking yourself if you really heard what they said, and are you responding to that or are you starting to tell them a story about yourself?

The communication battle is usually fought about who's not listening to who. Richard Carlson said in his best-selling book, *Don't Sweat The Small Stuff*, "By being the first person to reach out and listen, you stop the spiral of stubbornness". Maybe the foreign policy leaders of the world should take a few communication classes as well; it could save the world. If you don't make other people feel understood first, and instead try to cram your opinions down their throat, you will accomplish nothing. If you don't see someone else's side first, they will never see yours; even if they say that they agree with you, they're probably lying.

"A man convinced against his will is of the same opinion still" – Dale Carnegie

People who have mastered their mind think well, listen well, and as a result, they talk well. So when the time comes for you to open your mouth and speak, the most important thing you can do is paraphrase what the other person is trying to say. Now, like most things in life, there's good paraphrasing and there's bad paraphrasing. In the beginning, when I was first learning how to do this and was having trouble sounding like I really gave a crap about what the other person was saying, I would just repeat exactly what the other person said. But I believe that this is still better than totally disregarding what someone is saying so that I can talk about my point instead. It will also probably be obvious to the other person that you are paraphrasing, but this is also important because they will then know that at least you're making an effort, however small, to be a mirror for them and make them feel seen. With more practice, and as we experience the fruits of our communicating labor, we will get more creative with our paraphrasing as we also get better at genuinely caring about the other person's point of view. A relationship is like a quilt that over time get holes worn in it. Paraphrasing provides us with the needle, thread, and patches to keep everything together.

Not being understood by someone close to me is almost as painful as some sort of war torture. In fact, the military probably uses this tactic to illicit intelligence information from its captives. Obviously, I'm exaggerating here, but depending on how poorly our parents listened to us and empathized with us, not being heard can be extremely painful. If the house was on fire and I was trying to get someone close to me to understand that the house was on fire, but they didn't understand me, I would be almost as upset by the fact that they didn't understand me as I would be by the fact that we were all going to die in the fire. This is why I usually can't even remember why I got into a disagreement with them in the first place. The only thing I remember is that I was not heard. Fortunately, I've been able to become a better listener, which has had the paradoxical effect of improving the quality of understanding I receive in return. Being a good listener is contagious.

If I can narrow down the most common cause of disagreements, it's the moment when someone is trying to explain their issue to someone else, and the other person says, "I understand what you're saying, but ...", then they go off and talk about their own opinion. Or worse, they just cut you off without even acknowledging what you said altogether. When I first learned about this, I was shocked at how often I was doing this in my own relationships. Someone once said the following, and if you remember nothing else from this discussion, remember this: "Understanding is something that should be conveyed by the person who feels understood". In other words, if someone is trying to explain their position to you and they get frustrated because they don't feel like you understand them, and you keep saying, "I understand, I understand, but...", and then you try to explain your position, it doesn't matter what you say because the other person doesn't feel understood. You could be telling them where you buried a golden donkey, but if you didn't make them feel heard, THEY WON'T CARE! You have to get the other person to tell you or give you some indication that they feel understood, and this is accomplished by paraphrasing. By saying, "Let me get this straight because I want to understand you, what you're saying is ...", and if they say, "Yes, that's it!", then and only then do you have permission to move to the next level, which is discussing your own position.

The irony of this process is that by slowing the whole conversation down with paraphrasing, both sides are given more time to think about the issue, which creates a solution's favorite environment to reveal itself in. In the end, oftentimes, the answer was so obvious that both sides end up laughing at how narrow-minded they were both being.

Keep in mind that this is not a battle between two people, the goal is to uncover the truth and solve the problem. Both sides must help each other focus on the problem at hand. Bringing things up that happened in the past has to be off limits. There's enough work in dealing with present and future issues without having to add the weight of past baggage on top of it.

By listening, paraphrasing, and making the other person feel understood, you're channeling the flow of the conversation in a positive direction. So often people enter a disagreement preprogrammed to expect the other person not to listen, since no one ever listens to them anyway. By being the first person to reach out and listen, you're throwing the other person off balance. They never really expected you to listen to them, so now they're thinking, "Oh crap, you're listening to me, is what I'm saying accurate?" It forces them to reexamine exactly what they're saying. This simple technique often gets the other person to change their position without any more effort on your part, because they never put enough thought into their own position in the first place.

At the end of the day, you have to pick and choose your battles. Sometimes it's just easier to let people have their way this time, and save your resistance for a more important issue. It's also way too easy to get wrapped up in the ego and just wanting to be right because you have some weird insecurity about the person you're talking to (I used to do this all the time and still do sometimes). You think, "If I let them think they're right and I'm wrong, then they'll think they're better than me." Our caveman instincts make us want to fight to the death rather than admit we're wrong, but the question again is, "Do you want to be right, or do you want to be dead right?". It's not worth ruining a whole day or having a stroke just to win an argument. I spent my life using up enormous amounts of energy fighting for stupid little things that made no difference at all. One of the most amazing things that I've learned to do is to let people have their way when it really doesn't make a difference otherwise. It was a difficult battle with my ego for a while, because I always thought that I had a better and more efficient way to see and do things. I bit my tongue thousands of times, but now I just step aside and put my hand out, letting people have their way. I immediately let the resistance go and it feels so good; it's a powerful and exciting feeling to see how much control I have over myself now. It's like having a tug-of-war with someone, and then you just let go of the rope. The other person ends up flying across the room, and you can feel the release of tension; it's amazing. By unexpectedly letting people get their way, it often makes your viewpoint seem much more appealing to them, especially if they were insecure about their own opinion in the first place, which is often the case.

If all else fails with a breakdown in communication, we can resort back to Socrates and ask a simple question, "What do you want?". Posing this question to someone who's being difficult will redirect their focus from looking at the problem to looking at possible solutions. We should also pose this questions to ourselves when we're having a tug-of-war with ourselves in our own minds.

Some other indispensable communication tips that have helped me along the way are the following:

*No "F" bombs! It was hard to eliminate these from my heated discussions and it's still a work-in-progress. But they really are *bombs* in the sense that they destroy understanding rather than foster it. If you're feeling the need to swear, then perhaps taking a *time-out* to cool off is what's needed.

*Tone it down. This is another work-in-progress. It's hard to speak softly and slowly when you're enraged, but you'll be amazed at how effective it is. People can't hear what you're saying when you're yelling at them (except sometimes in an emergency). One of my favorite lines is from the movie, *The Interpreter*, starring Nicole Kidman and Sean Penn, about a planned assassination attempt on the president of an African country. The president is giving a speech to his people and states, "Even the lowest whisper can be heard over armies... when it's telling the truth", I still get goose bumps when I think about it. So try this the next time you're in a heated conversation: just lower your voice to almost a whisper and watch the look on people's faces. Making a powerful statement softly can make someone's hair stand up on end, whereas shouting at people just makes them deaf.

*Notice when you're getting amped up and de-escalate with some deep breaths. The more emotional you get, the less communication will take place.

*Say what you want, not what you don't want. You could go on forever complaining about what the problems are. The key is to focus on the solution, not the problem. Say what you want.

For me, this process of learning how to talk to people better was very much like trying to talk to someone in another language that I didn't know very well. I'm getting better at it, but it's challenging when so many other people don't know the language either. It's too bad this language isn't taught in school; maybe someday it will be. Until then, we have to teach ourselves, and then our spouses and children, the language of life. Without knowing how to talk to people, our relationships, our family, and our life will be a disaster. Living your life is kind of like flying an airplane, where you're the pilot, your spouse is the co-pilot, and the rest of your family are the other crew members. If you all suck at communicating, the plane's going down.

Face Facts

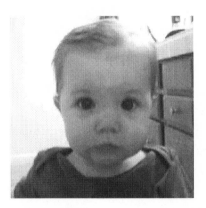

We know that to think, listen, and speak well is extremely important in maintaining a successful relationship, but what about mannerisms and facial expressions. It has been estimated that between 60% and 80% of all of our communication with other people is non-verbal, yet most of us have no idea what we look like when we talk to other people, and we don't even realize the vast amount of information we're sending with our face and body.

John Gottman is a professor in psychology at the University of Washington, and is known for his research on how married couples interact and handle disagreements. He has helped thousands of couples improve their relationships by helping them avoid hurtful behaviors. Several of Gottman's studies have shown significance in their ability to predict which couples will get divorced based on some simple observations of how they interact with each other. Gottman discovered that the behaviors that are most predictive of divorce are: criticism of a partner's personality, contempt, defensiveness, and emotional withdrawal or stonewalling.

Much of Gottman's research is based on videotaped interactions of couples. He scored them based on their behavior and linked their facial expressions to emotions such as disgust, contempt, anger, sadness, etc. For example, disgust is displayed by an ever so slight curling of the upper lip and scrunching the nose as if growling. These expressions are often barely noticeable if you're not paying attention, but after learning about all of this, I started catching myself making these expressions a lot when talking to people. Like when someone asks me a stupid question and I say, "What?!" with a look of disgust on my face. The problem is that every time we make these facial expressions to someone else, we're chipping away at the foundation of the relationship, especially if it's the person we've chosen to spend the rest of our life with.

Contempt is one of the most destructive emotions to express to your spouse, according to Gottman, and involves putting them down in some way. The facial expression of contempt is displayed by rolling one's eyes at the other person, or it is displayed by a half smile or pursing one half of the mouth and raising the other side. Again, I've found myself doing this regularly at work, especially when someone says something ignorant to me. Contempt is a secondary emotion, and a mix of the primary emotions disgust and anger.

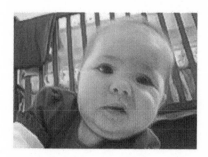

Gottman's models incorporate Paul Ekman's method of analyzing human emotion and microexpressions. Paul Ekman is a psychologist who has pioneered the study of emotions and their relationship to facial expressions. He has created an "atlas of emotions" with more than ten thousand facial expressions, and has been named one of the most influential people in the world by Time Magazine because of his research. Ekman found that our basic emotions are directly linked to our facial expressions, which are often involuntary because they happen before our conscious mind has time to become aware of the emotion behind the expressions. Ekman has also created fascinating training videos for police, government agencies, corporations, and medical professionals, to help them better understand their clients' true feelings. I watched one of his training videos and was amazed at how much awareness it brought to my daily interactions with other people. Some of the videos are just an hour long, and can teach you how to detect facial clues that last fractions of a second.

*

Libraries are filled with books written on non-verbal communication, which makes it even more interesting to consider how little we pay attention to it in ourselves and in others. The more I learn about it, the more fascinated I am with just watching people talk to me, and watching people talk to each other; it's like there's a whole other world that exists to me now. Some of the mannerisms are obvious, but you will be surprised at how often you can catch yourself doing them. Some of my favorites are: crossing your arms in front of you which can signal a defensive posture, unless of course you're just cold; then there's blinking your eyes frequently which can be a sign of lying, unless of course there's something stuck in your eye; poor eye contact is also a sign of being dishonest, unless you have an anxiety disorder like me, then you might find it uncomfortable to look someone in the eyes.

Ekman says that the face is an enormously rich source of information about what's going on inside our mind. His research has also found a link between our facial expressions and our nervous system, revealing that putting a smile on your face physically changes you for the better. I make myself smile all the time, especially when I don't feel good, because I know it will somehow make me feel better.

121

Being even just a little more aware of other people's nonverbal communication, as well as our own, gets us much closer to the truth of the messages being sent and received. Perhaps most importantly though, it makes us more aware of how often we make the people we love smile.

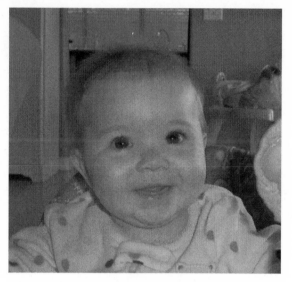

Keep It Alive

Most couples laugh a lot when they first get together, but after a while, things often aren't all that funny anymore. It takes some time, but once the dust settles, once you stop projecting yourself onto your partner and start seeing them for who they really are, and assuming you two are part of the fifty percent that still love each other and want to stay together forever, it's time to start laughing again. Then you'll remember why you two got together in the first place, because you *get* each other and you know what *that look* means. You'll also remember that you two are still together because your partner listened to you. They listened to you after they weren't listening to you for so long and you had a meltdown because of it, but then they listened; and for the first time in your life, when it mattered the most, someone really heard you, and it was the person you decided to spend the rest of your life with and you think, "Wow, did I get lucky", and you two start laughing again.

So many couples spend their time and energy raising their children and managing their careers that nothing is left to put into the relationship. What people don't realize is that, if the relationship falls apart, so does everything else. The relationship needs the same nurturing as a child does, so we have to make sure that it's also taken care of. Like a child needs things to be ever new and exciting, so do the adults in a relationship who get bored just as easily as children do.

Make sure you're always that couple in the restaurant who looks like they're on an awesome first date, the ones that are laughing a little too loud and covering their mouths so they don't get in trouble. Make sure you're not the couple that looks like they're on their way to a funeral - the funeral for their relationship because it's already dead.

Chapter 12

THE BODY IS A TEMPLE

It would be tragically ironic if you got to the point in your relationship with your spouse where everything is really good, no more fist fights, great sex, you two laugh all the time, and then one of you drops dead because you didn't physically take care of yourself. This book would not be complete without a discussion on how to treat your body like a temple. Your brain will work sluggishly at best, and you will not be able to master your mind, if you're treating your body like a garbage can. We're all aware of the basics - exercising and eating well, but there's so much more to it. The problem is that trying to weed through all of the information and studies out there is exhausting.

Despite all of my nursing education, I've still had to spend years researching this subject; beyond exercising and the decades-old food pyramid, nothing else is taught in nursing or medical school about how to really take care of yourself. Trying to figure out which vitamins and how much to take based on the conflicting information that's available was like trying to decipher heiroglyphics. I will summarize what I've learned and try to steer you in the right direction, but the decisions you make about your body are ultimately yours, and you must dedicate some time to do your own research, and consult your doctor before taking any new vitamins because everyone is different, and everything has side-effects.

*EXERCISE - this one's pretty easy; get off your ass and move more. I strive to get four days per week of 45 minutes of cardio, unless you have a bad heart then consult your doctor (I will make this statement throughout this book, but in other words, if you take any of my advice and then drop dead, don't try to blame it on me). For most of my life, I was exercising once or twice a week and patting myself on the back for this. Then I started getting older and becoming more aware of my own mortality - seeing people die every day helps in this area. I've always been afraid of getting cancer, so after doing a lot of research, I realized that I have the power to decrease cancerous growths by simply exercising more and eating healthy. I used to think that people either have cancer, or they don't. Then I learned that some people can have cancer in their body that either goes away or never becomes a problem, depending on how healthy their lifestyle is. So I've made exercise a central part of my life now.

I go out of town a lot, and I found that I couldn't exercise because I didn't have an elliptical or exercise bike to use on the road. I always told myself that I couldn't jog because I have bad knees, a bad back, and no stamina. One day I finally asked myself why I couldn't just try to jog, so I did, and I haven't stopped jogging since; my knees and back are fine by the way, and my stamina is better than it was in my twenties. I love to jog, and I can do it anywhere, anytime. I go very slow, so slow that my dog just walks by my side; she never even gets up to a trot. But my heart rate gets up to where it should be for my age and weight, and I use a cheap heart rate monitor on my wrist that I also love and highly recommend.

It's amazing how many excuses people have for why they can't do anything to make their lives better. They talk to me about their excuses all the time; it is as if they're trying to convince themselves that they're doing the right thing by not doing anything. The irony is that the energy they put into making excuses is more exhausting than exercising would be; I get exhausted just listening to them.

If I haven't convinced you yet that you should move more, then maybe this will change your mind. Most people have never heard of a pulmonary embolus or PE. It's a blood clot that usually forms in the deep veins of your legs (also known as a DVT or deep vein thrombosis) and travels to your lungs. The best way to get one of these things is to sit on the couch, or in the car, or in an airplane. As the flow of blood in your body starts to slow down due to your lack of movement, it has a tendency to start forming clots after about a half hour. Then, when you get up to go to the bathroom or go to the refrigerator, the blood clots dislodge from your leg and travel to your lungs. According to the Centers for Disease Control, as many as 900,000 people get DVT/PEs in the United States every year, and as many as 100,000 people die of them each year. Many die suddenly, and since up to forty percent of cases get missed, you may have a greater chance of dying from a pulmonary embolism than almost anything else. If this doesn't get you to exercise more, then the least you could do is something I like to call a *hipchuck*. A hipchuck is when you're in a sitting position and you thrust your hips forward and flex your legs and calves to increase the blood flow through your legs to prevent the formation of clots. Our family does a hipchuck every thirty minutes on all road and airplane trips. Richard Carlson, author of *Don't Sweat the Small Stuff* and who I have also quoted in this book, died of a pulmonary embolism at the age of 45 during a flight from San Francisco to New York while on a book tour.

*DIET - Stop cramming so much food in your mouth! I would never say this to anyone's face; it sounds terrible. But I think this to myself because I get angry and frustrated when I see my friends and loved ones who are overweight load their plates with too much food at the dinner table. I know, all too well, how they're slowly killing themselves with food, and I certainly don't want to lose them over such a preventable problem. Overeating is one of the few medical problems you can fix all by yourself, with your own hands. (Always consult with your doctor before making any dietary changes, especially if you're a diabetic and need to closely monitor blood sugar levels.)

I was also fascinated to find out that sugar substitutes can make people eat more. Based on a study done on rats, researchers discovered that eating sweet stuff with little or no calories sends a message to the brain telling it that we need to eat significantly more food in order to get enough calories to survive, so it has the effect of making us eat even more.

While you're trying to stay away from sugar substitutes, you may want to also cut down on your real sugar as well. One of my friends was telling me about her aunt who had breast cancer and how she cut out all of the added sugar in her diet. Then she said something that I'll never forget, "Cancer eats sugar". I almost fell of my chair; why hadn't anyone told me this before? Maybe I had been told that before, but no one ever said it like that. Anyway, I never before thought twice about cramming candy in my mouth. I always justified eating sweet stuff because I wasn't overweight and generally ate healthy, so I did a little research and found out about another study done on rats. The rats that were fed extra sugar, even more than the recommended daily allowance, got significantly more cancerous tumors than those that were on a low sugar diet. Now there's a lot of controversy about this, but I figured it wouldn't kill me to cut back a little on my sugar consumption. First I had to figure out how much daily sugar was acceptable, which took me a while, but 24 grams per day for a woman is what I came up with. Then I learned that one teaspoon of sugar equals four grams of sugar, so about 6 teaspoons was what I was allowed to have in a day. Using my astute math skills from high school, I realized that I was putting all of my daily sugar allowance in my morning coffee. "Great," I thought, "I'm gonna die!" After I checked my entire body for tumors, I calmed down and told myself that perhaps I could start out by putting a little less sugar in my coffee, and maybe only cram six peanut butter cups in my mouth, instead of the usual twelve.

Eating fruits and vegetables is a no-brainer, no pun intended, and some people believe that if your diet consisted of only organic fruits and vegetables you wouldn't get cancer at all.

There is also a growing number of foods and spices that show strong anti-cancer properties. Turmeric, which is the ingredient in mustard that makes it yellow, is at the top of the list. It doesn't taste that great but it's easy to disguise and I try to put it in everything; I think I've heard more positive anti-cancer effects of this spice than any other (it's best absorbed with some black pepper). All berries in general have strong antioxidant properties, especially blueberries. Green tea is very high in antioxidants, and recent research has shown that cruciferous vegetables, those whose stem and body shape resembles a cross like broccoli, cauliflower, brussel sprouts, and bok choy have significant anti-cancer effects (cruciferous vegetables effect the thyroid so check with your doctor before consuming large amounts them; also, cooking cruciferous vegetables decreases their effect on the thyroid).

The bottom line is that if you're eating this powerful stuff every day, and trying to avoid the bad stuff, your brain and body are going to be in a lot better shape than the person next to you that's eating deep-fried battered cake sticks at the county fair.

*HORMONES – While I was on my crusade to do everything humanly possible to avoid getting cancer, I stumbled upon a fascinating book that changed my life called, *Your Life In Your Hands*, by Professor Jane Plant. After reviewing all of her research, I was convinced that foods that have animal hormones in them are putting me at risk of getting cancer. Trying to completely eliminate them was extremely difficult, so I try to avoid them as much as possible. I also believe that the synthetic hormone-like chemicals found in some plastics are pro-cancerous, so I try to avoid them as much as possible by using stainless steel and ceramic containers. The vast majority of people at work microwave their food in plastic containers, especially the cute soft plastic containers that most TV dinners come in. "Hello! You're melting the plastic into your food and then eating it, are you sure you want to do that?"

*VITAMINS - This is a controversial topic and has always been since the days of snake oil. Some say it's a scam; some say it's not. Some studies say supplements make people healthier, some say they don't. It's very confusing even for me, so don't feel bad if you're confused about it. I have always taken vitamins ever since my mother handed me my first *One-A-Day* vitamin with a cigarette in her hand. My uncle is 92 years old and swears by them. At this point, it would be hard for anyone to convince me that I don't need to take vitamins. In school, we had to record everything we ate for two weeks, and then break down everything and figure out how much of each vitamin and nutrient we were getting. I was shocked to see how deficient I was in every category.

Choosing which vitamins to take and how much can be daunting. There are thousands of different brands of multivitamins and they all have different amounts of everything. To make it easier on myself, I had to find a good source for my information and choices, so I decided to go with Dr. Andrew Weil. Dr. Weil is the most reputable holistic doctor I know of, with degrees in medicine and biology from Harvard, and he's the director of the Arizona Center for Integrative Medicine at the University of Arizona. Dr. Weil's website, drweil.com, offers one of the best arrays of vitamin and health information that I've ever found, as well as a *vitamin advisor* which gives personalized suggestions on what supplements to take, as well as dosages.

*RADIATION EXPOSURE - Somewhere along the way, the catastrophizer in me became fascinated with environmental sources of radiation exposure, coupled with my fear of getting cancer. It's amazing to me how most people aren't very concerned about this. Radiation is everywhere; it's in certain foods, in the air, and in our homes. If we want to live a long and healthy life then we need to avoid radiation as much as possible. I could write a book about this subject alone, but I'll just list some main sources for now.

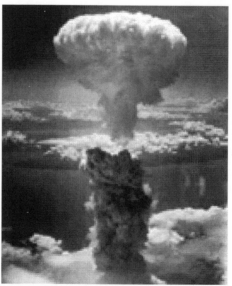

Did you know that one in fifteen houses has unacceptably high levels of radioactive radon gas in it, and that radon gas is the second leading cause of lung cancer after cigarette smoking? You can check your home's level by going to epa.gov and purchasing a cheap test kit. When you buy a house, there's no requirement to check for radon, so you're kind of playing Russian Roulette, unless you specifically ask for the house to be tested before you buy it. Fortunately, my house has acceptably low levels of radon, which is a naturally occurring gas that seeps out of cracks in the ground and sometimes gets stuck in your house. If you find you have high levels, you can retrofit your house with special vents which can cost a few thousand dollars, but at least you won't die from the radon. Also, your beautiful granite counter tops can be more radioactive than regular stone due to bits of uranium that naturally occur in granite; the uranium also gives off radon gas as well. After a water leak in our house, we had to redo the entire kitchen, and the first thing we did was rip out our granite countertops and replace them with beautiful wooden butcher block ones; they're gorgeous and we'll never have granite again. Hopefully we started a new trend. It's hard to believe how insistent people are to have radioactive granite in their homes.

If you're a hypochondriac and go to the doctor all the time, you probably get lots of x-rays and perhaps a few CT scans; lots of radiation here so try to avoid these unless absolutely necessary; fyi - MRIs are not radioactive, they're just more expensive so they're not always covered by insurance companies. I'm not very popular at my dentist office because I refuse to have x-rays done unless I'm having a problem, which is rare. I haven't had a complete set of x-rays done on my teeth in twenty years and nothing has been missed, yet they always try to make me feel bad about it, almost to the point of harassing me. I think dental insurance covers one or two complete sets of x-rays a year, which, over a life-time adds up to a bit of radiation exposure. I take care of people with brain tumors every day and I can't help but wonder if a life-time of dental x-rays twice a year is a contributing factor. Unless you have bad teeth to begin with and don't take care of them, I believe x-rays this often are totally unnecessary if you brush and floss daily, but I'm sure most dentists in the country will disagree with me. Ultimately, the decision is yours to make.

Airport security has become another source of radiation with their new body scanners that claim to deliver "very small" doses of radiation. Everyone was outraged at the detail of one's body that these scanners revealed, but no one seemed to care about being irradiated. Can you imagine the exposure that people who travel all the time get over a lifetime? Fortunately, you can "opt-out" of the body scanner and get a pat-down instead. Every time I fly, I have to give myself extra time to deal with the pat-down procedure which is quite inconvenient. I often feel like a criminal by opting out because there's no special line for me, so I have to raise my hand and say, "I'd like to opt out!" in front of everyone, and it seems to throw everyone off. After the TSA agent pats you down in front of everyone, they put the gloves they used on you into a bomb sniffing machine. I never considered the potential that the gloves used on me would ever trigger a false-positive reading on the "she's got a bomb" machine, but one time when I opted out, I got one. I saw the TSA agent put her gloves in the machine like she always does. But then I realized that it was taking longer than usual to get the green light. Then the TSA agent spoke into her radio calling for back up. I knew I was in trouble then. My heart started beating out of my chest; I felt like a terrorist, and everyone at this point thought I might actually be one. As the crowd of TSA agents ascended upon me, no one explained anything to me except for, "Come with us". As I considered my options, I also considered the possibility that instead of getting on my airplane I might be spending the night in a federal prison in Cuba. I held my breath and desperately wondered what would happen next. Then they took me into a "special room" with more boxes of gloves, and I was praying to God that I wouldn't have to be stripped searched. Still, no one was talking to me. I was afraid to speak because I have no filters and I was afraid I would accidentally say the word "bomb". "Now what are you going to do?", I said in a quivering voice. "We're going to pat you down again", the manly girl said in a gruff voice. It seemed to me that if I set the bomb detector off once, it was likely to happen again. Now I was totally catastrophizing in my head. I felt like I was in North Korea and that if I set the alarm off again, I would be taken away to a far-off prison camp, never to be seen again. The machine gave me a green light, and they told me I was free to go, so I'll never know what would have happened. I've opted out many times since then and everything worked out fine, but give yourself a little extra time if you do opt-out.

Getting back to radiation exposure, I'm not sure what part of the world you live in, but in my area there are a few nuclear waste dumps. I found this out by stumbling upon the EPA's superfund site map. "What's a superfund site?", you ask. Well, it's a cute name that often refers to a toxic or nuclear waste dump. Apparently, they're all over the country, so you might want to make sure you don't live next to one. The reason I was looking into this was because I was concerned about the quality of my drinking water. Since I'm so worried about getting cancer, I wanted to make sure that I wasn't drinking water that had uranium in it, but apparently I was. Did you know that the EPA has set acceptable levels of uranium in drinking water? It's thirty micrograms per liter, which isn't very much, but for Christ's sake, it's uranium!! Anyway, to make a long story short, I found out that the only way to get uranium and 98% of all other contaminants out of my water was by either distilling the water, which can be costly, or by using a water filter that performs reverse osmosis. In my opinion, those cute little water filters in your refrigerator are a joke, an expensive joke. Most bottled water is tap water ran through reverse osmosis filters, and it usually says this on the label in the back. I got my water filter from freedrinkingwater.com for under $300, but they also started selling them at hardware stores. Uranium is probably not very good for your brain either, so if you're going to go through all the trouble to master your mind, you'll probably want to live as long as you can to use your new-found powers. Acceptable levels of anything that can kill you is not acceptable, so filter your drinking water properly.

The Children

It's a blessing that my daughter does not have any problems like autism or attention deficit hyperactivity disorder, also known as ADHD. But I was shocked to learn how common these two disorders are becoming. A new study by the CDC found a thirty percent increase in autism spectrum disorder, or ASD. Autism spectrum disorder (ASD) is a group of developmental disabilities that can cause significant social, communication and behavioral challenges. The study was an estimate based on eight-year-old children living in eleven different communities across the country. If you're planning on having a child today, this study found that about 1 in 68 of them will be identified with autism. The number of children identified with autism varied widely by community, from 1 in 175 children in areas of Alabama, to 1 in 45 children in areas of New Jersey.

According to the CDC, a person with ASD might:

Not respond to their name by 12 months of age
Not point at objects to show interest (point at an airplane flying over) by 14 months
Not play "pretend" games (pretend to "feed" a doll) by 18 months
Avoid eye contact and want to be alone
Have trouble understanding other people's feelings or talking about their own feelings
Have delayed speech and language skills
Repeat words or phrases over and over (echolalia)
Give unrelated answers to questions
Get upset by minor changes
Have obsessive interests
Flap their hands, rock their body, or spin in circles
Have unusual reactions to the way things sound, smell, taste, look, or feel

Attention deficit hyperactivity disorder, or ADHD, is another neurobehavioral disorder of childhood characterized by inattention, hyperactivity, disruptive behavior, and impulsivity. According to the CDC, recent surveys asked parents whether their child received an ADHD diagnosis from a health care provider. The results showed that approximately 11% of children 4-17 years of age, or 6.4 million children, have been diagnosed with ADHD. There has been an 11% increase in the incidence of ADHD in the last eight years, and the prevalence varies by state, from a low of 5.6% in Nevada to a high of 18.7% in Kentucky. Over 6% of children are taking medication for ADHD.

Children with ADHD may:

Get distracted easily and forget things often
Switch too quickly from one activity to the next

Have trouble with directions

Daydream too much

Have trouble finishing tasks like homework or chores

Lose toys, books, and school supplies often

Fidget and squirm a lot

Talk nonstop and interrupt people

Run around a lot

Touch and play with everything they see

Be very impatient

Blurt out inappropriate comments

Have trouble controlling their emotions.

Hmmm, the above list sounds like most of the children I know, and when I look at it I also think, "Wow, maybe I have ADHD," but I don't. So keep in mind that these behaviors should happen a lot and be quite disruptive to the children's life to meet the criteria.

The CDC goes on to say that data from international samples suggest young people with high levels of attentional difficulties are at greater risk of involvement in a motor vehicle crash, drinking and driving, and traffic violations. This no doubt contributes to the staggering "cost of illness" which, using a prevalence rate of 5%, estimates the cost to be between $36 and $52 billion dollars.

The amount of money we spend on these disorders is outrageous, but the benefit of preventing someone's life from being hurt by these disorders is priceless. The first question we have to answer is why are these disorders increasing at such an alarming rate? We must be doing something wrong. A large part of the problem seems to be genetic, but a significant influence is also from our environment. Mastering our minds includes helping our children master their own minds, which is even harder to do if the deck is stacked against them with these disorders. This is why it's so important to make sure that our environments and our children's environments are peaceful, loving, structured, focused, and not over or under-stimulated. They must also be free of as many chemicals and radioactive particles as possible - the ones in the air and the ones in our food and water.

You also may want to make sure that there's not a nuclear waste dump in your back yard. One of the biggest ones is in Hanford, Washington, where there are 177 enormous tanks being stored underground that contain about 50 million gallons of radioactive and chemical waste left over from the Manhattan Project; glad we don't live there. One of my family members lives in a suburb of Chicago and got lymphoma a few years ago. She's in remission now, thank God, but I remember before she got sick that her town mailed out letters warning them not to drink the water; it didn't say why though. Then I found out that the first nuclear reactor that was ever built in this country sat on a plot of land in her town, right down the road from her house, in a cute little forest preserve called Red Gate Woods, on the corner of 95th and Archer Avenue. This was where Albert Einstein and Enrico Fermi worked on the Manhattan Project. After the war was over and the government didn't need the reactor anymore, they dug a hole and pushed the entire reactor in the ground and swept some dirt on top of it. There it sits to this day, with a forest preserve and a bicycle path on top of it. There's also a cute monument on top that warns people not to dig there; it says at the bottom, "THERE IS NO DANGER TO VISITORS," but someone tried to erase the "NO" by carving it out of the stone as you can see in the picture.

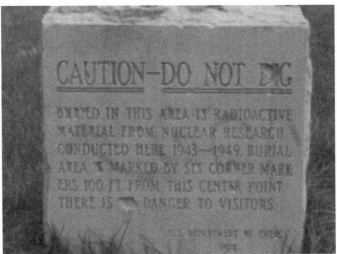

No one knows for sure if this had anything to do with my relative's lymphoma, but would you think you might get sick if there was a nuclear reactor buried in your neighborhood? I was unable to determine if there was a higher incidence of autism and ADHD in that area, but I wouldn't be surprised. In New Jersey, where the incidence of autism was found to be 1 child in 45, there are 149 Superfund sites listed on the EPA's list of most contaminated sites, in Alabama where the incidence of autism is 1 in 175 children, there are 18. In defense of New Jersey, the rate of ADHD there is low at only 5.5%, whereas Kentucky, with only 20 Superfund sites on the National Priority List, has the highest rate of ADHD at 18.7%, so there are other factors in play.

Chapter 13

HUMOR

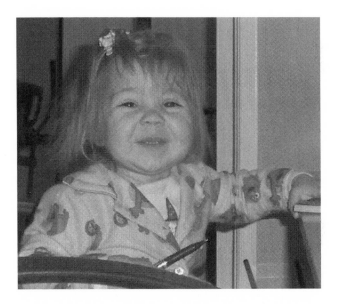

Now, enough about all this serious stuff, let's have a little fun, shall we? Do you think I'm funny? I think I'm funny, funny-looking, ha, ha, ha!! I laugh at myself all the time, but I haven't always been this hilarious. I used to be attracted to people who were funny, thinking that they were just born that way with some magical powers, and that I was cursed with the inability to tell jokes well and bad timing. I figured out that I could cultivate my sense of humor over time and learn how to do it from other funny people. So if you don't have a sense of humor, it's never too late to try and get one. I don't know what I would do without my sense of humor now. It has become one of my greatest assets, for myself and my family, and it's saved my life on several occasions - when I would have otherwise had a stroke from rage. Finding a thread of humor in difficult situations can derail the amygdala's attempt to make you freak out, and according to a study of over 100,000 people conducted by the National Institutes of Health, being funny is number two on the list of preferred traits of mates, number one is intelligence. So being smart and funny should guarantee you a mate for life.

Besides being smart, being funny is also one of the most important human attributes that can improve health in a broad spectrum of categories; and if you're funny, it also means that you're pretty smart too. The National Institutes of Health found that, "Humor involves the ability to detect incongruous ideas violating social rules and norms...and requires a complex array of cognitive skills for which intact frontal lobe functioning is critical." According to this, it seems that being funny is also the equivalent of mental gymnastics.

Several studies have shown that laughter significantly improves one's overall state of health and well-being; even if it's fake laughter, the body doesn't know the difference. Some studies have also shown that laughing significantly improves creativity, memory recall, and intelligence.

Brain scans done on people who are made to laugh show that the reward centers of the brain light up in response to this; it's like a mental jackpot. Some people with damage to the frontal lobe of their brain can't get jokes at all; it seems I've known several people with this problem. Research has also shown that the therapeutic effect of laughter is the same whether you make yourself laugh, or someone else does, the brain cannot tell the difference. Knowing this, I try to make myself laugh, as well as laugh at myself, as much as possible.

There are even people who claim that laughing cured their cancer, and they just may be right. More serious studies need to be done to prove this link, but I'm not going to wait for them. Like antibiotics, laughing hasn't been very profitable for the drugs companies, so I'm not sure how much research will be done in either area. In the meantime, I will try not to get an infection, unless it's from contagious laughter. Laughing is at the top of my list of life priorities, and my goal is to wake up each morning with a smile on my face, and go to bed laughing each night.

One of the keys to humor is creativity. People who are hilarious are also quite creative, so perhaps learning how to be more creative will bring more laughter into our lives. If all else fails, you could just smoke pot.

Chapter 14

CREATIVITY

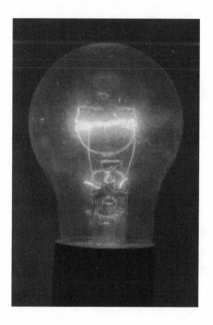

"Talent hits a target no one else can hit, genius hits a target no one else can see" -Arthur Schopenhauer, German Philosopher

Creativity requires something called bisociation, which means to make a connection between two or more completely different frames of reference, blending them together into a new meaning. A simple example of bisociation is when someone makes a pun or a joke, they use the element of surprise by connecting two totally different lines of thought, creating a eureka moment of sudden understanding, which can be very funny. Being funny is perhaps the best example of being creative, but the most important scientific discoveries of mankind also owe their evolution to creativity.

There has always been something divine about creative people. For centuries, creativity was believed to be a gift solely from the gods. It wasn't until the Renaissance, one of the most creative periods in human history, that mere mortals started getting some credit for their abilities. Somewhere along the way, perhaps during the American Revolution, the value of creativity started to fade. This may be in part due to the erroneous habit of viewing creative abilities as something that can't be scientifically explained, thereby eliminating it as a characteristic of genius. As a result, creative attributes became much less valued compared to the "left-sided brain" abilities of computing, memorizing, and calculating. Music, drama, and the arts have always taken a back seat to math and science, as is evidenced by the dramatic pay differences in these opposing fields. As such, most of us have been encouraged by our parents, like the Little Prince was, not to dilly-dally in the arts, but to spend our time planning and calculating.

Fortunately, there's been an uptick in interest in creativity as of late, maybe because of Sir Ken Robinson's TED talk on how schools kill creativity in children, the most viewed TED talk of all time. Perhaps it's due to the fact that people are beginning to realize how lucrative creativity can be. In a survey conducted by IBM of over 1500 CEOs from all over the world, the trait considered to be the most important for success and leadership was creativity.

People who are creative are more interesting, more successful, and generally happier than people who aren't. But the question is, how can we cultivate more creativity in our own lives, and how do creative people's brains work differently from those who aren't?

The concept of bisociation was first introduced by Arthur Koestler in his 1964 book, *The Act of Creation*. Koestler believed that many people's creativity is "...frequently suppressed by the automatic routines of thought and behavior that dominate their lives." His book also discusses how "people are most creative when rational thought is suspended." In other words, when we're relaxed and when we least expect it.

Perhaps we should first look at what's going on inside our brains when we're being creative. We already know that the right hemisphere is involved in making distant connections to different aspects of a problem, as opposed to the left brain which is associated with finding answers rationally and methodically, step by step. But as noted in Jonah Lehrer's fascinating book on creativity, *Imagine: How Creativity Works,* it wasn't until recently that the scientific community realized that the right hemisphere had any value at all. Now we're beginning to see how crucially important the right hemisphere is to our overall functioning, and especially to our creativity. Whereas the left hemisphere helps us see the trees, the right hemisphere gives us a better view of the whole forest, and one of the ways it does this is by giving us the ability to think divergently.

In general, there are two different kinds of thinking referred to as divergent thinking (right brain) and convergent thinking (left brain). Divergent thinking explores many different possible solutions, while convergent thinking follows a step-by-step formula to arrive at one solution. For example, if your car breaks down and you're mainly a convergent thinker, you think "I have to get to work without my car, how can I get there?" You're narrowly focused on getting to work, so you mathematically figure out that you can get your things together, walk to the bus stop and take the bus. Now you pat yourself on the back for coming up with the solution, because you assumed that there was only one option and one solution. But had you used some divergent thinking, you may have considered not even going to work that day, or perhaps you could have worked from home and conducted your appointments over the phone. Divergent thinking considers many different possible solutions, allowing sometimes unexpected outcomes. Once a solution is arrived at divergently, convergent thinking is effective at determining step-by-step how to make it happen, but if relied on solely, convergent thinking can get us stuck on a one-way street. This is also where challenging our thoughts by asking the right questions comes in to play as well. "What if I don't go to work today, what's the worst that will happen, and can I make something even better come out of it?" If you don't really like your job and you've been meaning to look for a new one, perhaps taking the day off to do so would change the entire course of your life.

People tend to use one strategy over the other to solve problems without even realizing it. But wouldn't the ideal situation be to increase our awareness and control our consciousness so that we choose which strategy to use, depending on what the problem at hand calls for, or perhaps to use each strategy together by varying degrees to maximize our ability to come up with the best solution?

Some of the most famous people in history were quite good at combining both types of thinking and problem solving, and by doing so, they changed the course of history with their discoveries. Isaac Newton's creative leap in discovering the law of gravity when he saw an apple fall from a tree is one example. Albert Einstein, after struggling for years to find an answer, suddenly had the solution to the general theory of relativity revealed to him in a daydream, stating that, "Like a giant die making an indelible impress, a huge map of the universe outlined itself in one clear vision." Charles Darwin spent much of his time creatively daydreaming, being accused by his father of being "lazy and too dreamy." So taking time to step out of your office and relax a bit can be worth its weight in gold.

*

Another pioneer of creativity was Graham Wallas, who wrote *Art of Thought*, published in 1926, which presented one of the first models of the creative process consisting of four stages:

Preparation - this is where the mind consciously gathers the information and plans the basic steps to complete the project or solve the problem.

Incubation - this is the period where there is somewhat of a break taken from narrowly focusing on the problem, but it is still being actively processed unconsciously, thus creating an opportunity for many different pieces of information to contribute to the solution.

143

Illumination - this is the moment when the conception of an idea, or the solution to a problem takes place. It moves from unconscious, to preconscious, to consciousness, and is experienced as an almost overwhelming flash of insight when the hair stands up on the back of your neck and you get goose bumps.

Verification - this is where the idea is consciously validated and where convergent thinking turns this abstract idea into something tangible.

Of these five steps, incubation is perhaps the most important because without it, it will be difficult for the birth of a creative solution to take place. If we can't find an answer to a problem, sometimes it's best to put it on the back burner and let it simmer for a while. It's often hard to let go of something that you've been holding on to so tightly, but if you loosen your grip a little and the conditions are just right, amazing things can happen.

Incubation involves a period of interruption or rest from a problem, which helps us avoid becoming fixated on overanalyzing the problem. Relying on convergent thinking to problem solve often leads to insanely going down the same "logical" brain pathways over and over again, without ever finding a solution. Creative solutions to difficult problems are often found some place you haven't looked before, and at a time when your thoughts travel down a different path and end up some place new.

*

It's unfortunate that some people who have amazingly creative ideas are often misunderstood or looked upon with contempt by others. Robert Goddard, quite possibly the greatest rocket scientist that ever lived, had his ideas "rejected and mocked by his peers who thought they were outrageous and impossible." Leonardo Da Vinci's ideas were so ahead of his time that many of them were not put to use until hundreds of years later. It has been said that it's human nature to destroy what one cannot understand, and creative ideas are often quite unusual and difficult to understand or visualize for people who are narrow-minded and perhaps not very creative themselves.

144

Sometimes, creative people are accused of being crazy. In fact, there seems to be a strong link between mood disorders and creativity, with one study finding an 80% correlation between the two. Writers, poets, and artists are at the top of the list of creative people who have mood disorders. Another study gave writers a suicide rate almost twice that of the general population. "Great!" I thought to myself, I finally found a new career and I'm going to kill myself anyway. There's certainly no shortage of amazingly creative people who have killed themselves. Vincent Van Gogh, Ernest Hemingway, and Robin Williams are but a few on a very sad and unbelievably long list. The implication here is that there's a fine line between genius and insanity; all the more reason to learn how to get control over the chaos in our minds and perhaps turn our creativity into something amazing. In the words of Casey Kasem, as long as we "keep our feet on the ground, we can keep reaching for the stars."

*

Let's talk some more about what's happening in our brains when we're being creative. We already know that the right side of the brain is where creativity evolves, but what exactly is happening here? There are five main types of brain waves that occur at different levels of consciousness, and what the latest research has shown is that an increase in alpha brain wave activity leads to an increase in creative thinking. Everything that's going on in our head results in electrical impulses that can be viewed on an EEG machine as waves.

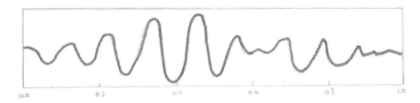

Alpha waves, so called because they were the first waves discovered, are present when your brain is in a relaxed state and not focused on any one particular thing. Creating alpha wave states is even being used to treat anxiety and depression, by teaching people to relax and ignore their unwanted thoughts. It turns out that this relaxed state is also the

145

perfect environment to have a creative insight, and people who have low levels of alpha wave activity find it harder to relax and be creative. Perhaps this explains why some people never get it, they just can't seem to figure out a solution to their problems. They never create an environment in their own lives that fosters alpha wave production in their minds, so they're never able to have insights into their own problems. We should be doing everything we can to enhance our surroundings to promote alpha waves, to promote relaxed, creative thought. Take a nice warm bath, light some candles, play some smooth jazz. Meditation is at the top of the list of things we can do to create alpha waves in our mind. Even meditating for just for a few minutes can do the trick, and you can do that anytime, any place.

Another thing we can do to increase our creativity is to put ourselves in a different place, mentally, physically, or both. Albert Einstein famously said that you can't solve a problem on the same level you were on when it was created. One way to get yourself on a different level is to just get out of the house or office for a little while, which can put everything in a new perspective. Getting in the car and going for a drive can put a whole new look on things. Taking a walk in the woods is one of my favorites, and while you're walking you might consider jogging or biking because there's also quite a bit of research out there linking exercise with creativity.

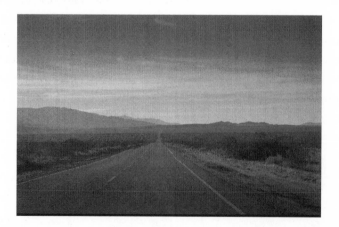

Surrounding yourself with certain colors can also have a significant effect on your creative abilities. A study conducted by the University of British Columbia set out to find which color, red or blue, improves brain performance and receptivity to advertising. It found that they both can, but while red was the most effective at enhancing our attention to detail, blue was the best at boosting our ability to think creatively. Based on this, I decided to paint my office blue. I've been analytically using the left side of my brain most of my adult life, so I decided that it's time to start using the other part of my brain. There are a few red accents though.

So who cares if we're more creative? Wouldn't it just be easier to sit on the couch and watch other people be creative? Of course it would be easier, but *easy* is boring, and we want to be more creative because it's really fun and stimulating for our brain. We're getting high on life by using our own minds instead of doing drugs or alcohol, and it's way better because there's no hangover or side-effects. We're not frying our brain - we're creating more brain cells. Having a eureka moment stimulates the pleasure centers of the brain, and it's addicting. It also feeds on itself. The more creative we are, the more creative we're going to be, and nothing is more rewarding and stimulating than creating something new with our unadulterated mind. But be careful not to feel too good about what you're doing or you could have a problem, like the rats in the brain experiments conducted in the 1950s. Researchers created a situation where the rats were able to directly stimulate the pleasure centers of their brain by pressing a lever. Once the rats discovered the lever, they chose to forgo food and sex in favor of pressing the lever, ultimately exhausting and starving themselves to death. The poor lifeless bodies of the little rats were found crumpled up in little balls on the floor beneath the levers. The scientists didn't have to torture and kill these poor rats though, they could have instead conducted their research on humans at a casino.

When we're having a rough time, we'll know we're headed back on track when we easily make ourselves feel good from within, without using drugs or alcohol, or a casino. When we feel bad, it's because there's a problem that needs to be solved, which in and of itself presents the best opportunity to have a creative breakthrough. If every problem is approached this way, then life will be transformed, and everything we do can be enjoyable.

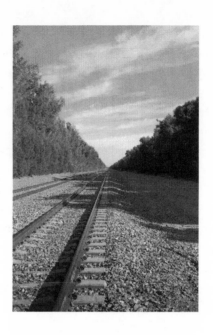

*

I finally realized that a good part of my unhappiness in life could be attributed to my anal-retentive and rigid compulsion to stick to a predetermined plan in everything that I did. Because of my low self-esteem, which I compensated for by trying to obsessively control everything, I decided that this was the best way to live my life, and that any deviation from this structure was just bad. Convergent thinking ruled my life. Fortunately, and better late than never, I changed my ways. At first, it was very difficult to deviate from my plans, or not even make plans at all. But soon I found it quite enjoyable to be spontaneous. Of course, I had to create a sort of litmus test in my mind to apply to each situation that I considered being spontaneous with. It's just a quick mental check that I do that gives my brain permission to let the plan go, but it works well; my stress levels have fallen significantly as a result, and I'm much more creative now. It's also hard to talk myself out of doing things now because before, if I didn't know exactly how something was going to go from beginning to end, I wouldn't do it out of fear of the unknown. It was perfect because it allowed me to talk myself out of just about anything that involved too much work or too much risk. What I didn't realize is that I was talking myself out of living my life by playing it safe, which is what many people end up doing. Creativity requires that we step out into the unknown.

One of my favorite analogies about living life with uncertainty is that of driving a car at night on a winding country road without a GPS navigation system, if anyone can remember what that's like. You can't see the entire road laid out before you, you can only see as far as your headlights are shining, but that doesn't stop you because you want to get to where you're going. You have faith in the fact that the road will not lead you off a cliff, and that if you follow the speed limit and street signs, you'll make it to where you want to go safely. It's impossible to know exactly what turns lie ahead because you've never been on this road before. You can do your research, but at some point, you're going to have to have faith that things will unfold in a reasonable manner, so you can keep moving forward, being cautiously optimistic, and perhaps at some point you can even sit back and enjoy the ride.

Chapter 15

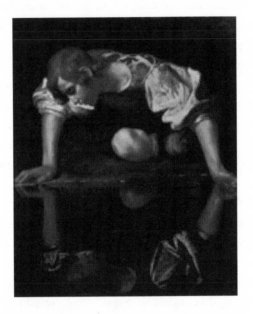

"Narcissus falls in love with his own image, but he doesn't know it is he that is loved" -Thomas Moore

As we journey into the unknown, our greatest companion who will be motivating us and making us feel safe will be our Self, or our self-esteem. Some people have been taught that self-love is bad, and that the goal should be to give ourselves to others until there is nothing left to give. Then, if there's anything left of ourselves, we can love that a little, but not too much. Others have been taught that it's all about themselves, that if they're not happy then no one should be happy, and that they should get a medal just for participating. Some people mistakenly call this high self-esteem. The problem lies in understanding the definition of healthy vs. unhealthy self-love, or high self-esteem vs. low self-esteem.

Narcissists are fascinating people and they give us perhaps the best example of what unhealthy self-love and low self-esteem looks like. Contrary to popular belief, narcissists do not really love themselves at all; in fact, some would say they despise themselves. But the irony is that if they loved themselves for who they are, and accepted all of the good and the bad within them, then they would see how beautiful they really are. Instead, narcissists are caught in a masquerade of constantly trying to hide their imperfections and prove that they're the most amazing people in the world, even though they know, deep down inside, that nothing could be further from the truth.

I never knew how much I disliked myself until I started reading books on self-esteem. I always thought that I loved myself; I mean, doesn't everybody think that? But the more I read, the more I realized that I had quite a bit of work to do in the area of self-acceptance. It was also interesting to see how others around me didn't like themselves all that much either.

If you want to know everything there is to know about self-esteem, the foremost expert on the subject is Nathaniel Branden. In his book, *The Six Pillars of Self-Esteem*, Dr. Branden defined self-esteem as "confidence in our ability to cope with the basic challenges of life" and "confidence in our right to be successful and happy". Many of us have low self-esteem, so if a problem arises in our life and we freak out about it, we're freaking out because we don't think we can handle it, and we also think that success and happiness only happen to people who deserve it, but not to us. So we set our expectations for life low enough to ensure that we will never have to suffer a failure, or that we will never receive anything too amazing that we don't think we deserve. In the end, we usually get what we expect.

People with healthy levels of self-esteem set their standards for what they think is acceptable, in all areas of their life, high enough to guarantee them a certain degree of happiness. But unlike narcissists who destructively and self-indulgently demand immediate gratification from little or no effort on their part, people with high self-esteem have a desire to get the most out of life that is in harmony with everything and everyone around them, and they are often willing to go to the ends of the earth to get it.

According to Dr. Branden, one word that captures the essence of self-esteem is perseverance. Perseverance is the quality in someone that motivates them to continue trying to finish something even though it is very difficult, when others would just give up. People with high self-esteem don't let their own lack of knowledge stand in their way. If they don't understand something, they look for answers when most people would give up the search for the truth, and simply avoid all unknowns like potential land-mines. Fortitude is another word that makes me think of people with high self-esteem. Fortuitous people have the strength to handle misfortune or discomfort with patience and calm.

Reacting calmly under stress is another attribute of people with high self-esteem. Working in an ICU, when a patient's heart stops beating, panicking is not an option for the nursing staff, and the calmer everyone is, the more likely it will be that we will save someone's life. But some people do panic, and it's unfortunate but interesting to see people's true colors in a life-threatening situation. I've always been pretty good at looking calm on the outside, but I used to panic inside all the time, and every now and then, I still do. In the ICU, we have digital screens that display our patient's vital signs so we can constantly monitor them. Many patients are very sick and on the verge of death all the time. Not many things could be more nerve-wracking than suddenly seeing your critically ill patient's heart rate and blood pressure on the display screen start to drop precipitously. While you desperately try and figure out if there's anything you can do to prevent them from flat-lining, you also know that you only have about ten seconds to figure it out before they die and you have to try and bring them back to life. My heart used to pound out of my chest every time this would happen, and I realized that if I didn't start to react more calmly, I was going to flat-line. I started using the Navy Seal amygdala control techniques and trained myself to not respond so physically and emotionally to these situations, and I instead used the frontal lobe of my brain more, coupled with some deep breathing. Now, my heart doesn't beat out of my chest every time my patient crashes, and I have a lot more control over the situation which is very empowering.

Besides reacting calmly under stress, people with high self-esteem also thrive on the unknown because they know that, like outer space and the physical universe, 99.9% of everything that can be known is still unknown, and that the only way to get from here to there is to plow through the uncertainty, continuously answering the questions that arise.

Learning how people of high self-esteem conduct their lives made me realize all of things that I was doing wrong in my life. Every time an unknown would arise, I would get stressed out over it and lose energy - precious energy that could have been used to just solve the problem. When something difficult came up that I was struggling with, it was a catastrophe, and I would always interpret my struggle as a direct reflection of my total incompetence as a human being. In my relationships with other people, if someone didn't like me, it was because I was a bad person, not because they were projecting their own self-hatred on me. If I liked someone a lot, it was because they were the most amazing person in the world, and of course they probably wouldn't want to be friends with someone as inferior as myself. I needed to get myself together, so I set out to learn how an ideal person acts and treats themselves and others, so I could be more like that. Ironically, the first thing that I needed to do was to cut myself some slack.

There are many things we can do to increase our self-esteem, but the most important things are cutting ourselves some slack when we fail, and cutting others some slack when they fail. Expecting ourselves and everyone else to be perfect is totally unrealistic and will leave us constantly disappointed. People with high self-esteem are masters at keeping their expectations low enough so that they spend most of their time pleased with the outcomes of their lives, while still maintaining forward momentum. On the other hand, people with low self-esteem are continuously disappointed with life, expend enormous amounts of energy running in circles, miss their own unrealistic goals regularly, and make very little progress. This was how I used to spend every day of my life.

While we're cutting ourselves some slack for failing, keeping our proudest accomplishments of life in mind is very motivating, especially during those times when we feel like complete failures. We also need to be well aware of exactly what we want to be spending our precious time doing. We cannot always do everything we want because there's just not enough time, and we want to be good at what we've chosen to do, so having perhaps three or four major things that we're involved in is best. We don't want to spread ourselves too thin because this is a common cause of anxiety. I have a vision board in my studio to inspire and remind me of the most important things that I want to spend my limited time here doing.

*

Some other attributes of people with high self-esteem are the following:

*They are able to talk about their accomplishments as well as their failures objectively, and without exaggeration, although I often exaggerate about my failures just because it's really funny and it makes me feel good to laugh at myself.
*They happily take compliments, instead of shooting them down because they don't think they deserve them. It's okay to just say thanks when someone compliments you. People with high self-esteem are also able to take criticism with dignity and accept and acknowledge their mistakes, as opposed to playing victim and blaming others for their problems, or erupting with defensive rage at each criticism.
*They are open to new ideas and new potentials for life, as opposed to rejecting anything new and having a fear of the unknown.
*They are able to laugh at themselves and generally see the humor in life every day, and they are able to see the humor in others harmlessly, and without inflicting wounds on others' self-esteem; they do not take joy in other people's pain but are able to empathize with them.
*They handle themselves well under stress without coming unglued because they know they can handle it.

154

*They have a generally positive outlook on life, and see setbacks as temporary rather than catastrophic.

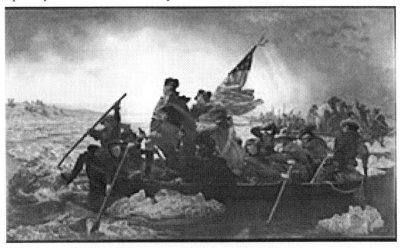

Washington crossing the Delaware

Mastering the mind requires maintaining a healthy level of self-esteem because without it, the door to chaos will be open. We must accept the good and the bad within ourselves, and remind ourselves that even the most amazing people have faults. If we commit to appreciating the good in ourselves, and improving and overcoming the bad, we will learn to love ourselves, perhaps for the first time in our lives, and we will make it easier for others to love us.

Projection

Carl Jung viewed the Self as an internal force that guides us consciously and unconsciously, and that can only be fully grasped by interpreting our dreams. He considered the Self to be the central regulating force within us, that brings about growth and integration of different aspects of our personality. Jung called this integration of the personality individuation, and considered the spiritual picture of the Mandala as symbolizing this unification of our Self. If we fail to reach this level of individuation, and are unable to integrate all of the good and bad aspects of ourselves, then one of the fascinating things that can happen unconsciously is called projection. When someone is projecting, their unacceptable thoughts, impulses, and desires are dealt with by placing them outside of themselves, and attributing them to someone else. Narcissists are masters of projection.

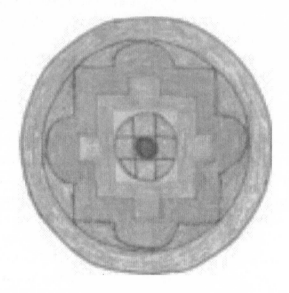

People with low self-esteem feel like they don't have any control over their lives, so turning an internal threat (feeling ignorant about something) into an external threat (accusing someone else of being ignorant), gives them a false sense of control over their own out-of-control lives. By raising our self-esteem, we can increase our awareness of times when we could be rejecting parts of our self, and projecting these parts onto someone else. When we have deep emotional responses to other people, whether good or bad, there's a chance that a projection is taking place, and it's helpful to consider this at the time.

Projection doesn't just involve our negative characteristics, it can involve a person seeing amazing qualities in another person that they don't realize they possess themselves. This often happens in codependent relationships where someone thinks another person is amazing and that they're not good enough for this other person. The truth is that we all project things from time to time, but there is a link between how low someone's self-esteem is and how much projection takes place. Being able to recognize those times when a projection is taking place will help us spot areas in our self or in others that need some work; it will give us more emotional control over our relationships.

There are many interesting examples of projection, such as accusing your spouse of having an affair, or being a bully. We've all heard of the typical scenario where one spouse is thinking about having an affair, and instead of accepting this reality, they accuse the other spouse of having an affair in order to relieve some of their own overwhelming guilt. When people feel guilty about something, they usually project whatever unacceptable behavior they've committed onto someone else by making false accusations. This temporarily relieves some of their anxiety over unacceptable feelings. There's also the example of the bully at school or work who projects their own vulnerability onto the person they're bullying to make themselves feel better about their own sense of fear and insecurity.

Projection can bring about some temporary relief from our own insecurities, but at the same time, it prevents us from having a whole, unified Self, as Carl Jung viewed as the purpose of life. We cannot truly have peace in our lives until this integration takes place. Depending on how low our self-esteem is, it could be a slow and painful process of acknowledging and accepting some often-unpleasant things about ourselves. Fortunately, there are usually some really good things that we, for whatever reason, have neglected to accept about ourselves that we also need to come to terms with. We could say to ourselves, "Wow, I really am a pretty cool person after all." Or, "I guess I'm smarter than I thought I was", or "Wow, I guess I really can make a difference." There's always some good to take with the bad.

As far as intimate relationships go, we are able to love our partners more deeply when our projections are removed and we see the person as they really are. But sometimes the opposite occurs and we realize that who we "fell in love" with is not the person we thought they were; then the relationship falls apart because our partner is not nearly as amazing as we projected them to be. Most of my relationships ended this way with me saying, "What was I thinking?" Now I know what I was thinking, and arming myself with this knowledge has become a powerful tool for my mind, and has allowed me to finally have the real and lasting relationship that I always hoped to find.

Codependence/Reparenting

A discussion about getting our Selves together would not be complete without mentioning codependence. Being codependent is another side-effect of low self-esteem. Most of us have heard of this disorder from Alcoholics Anonymous, where the term is used to refer to someone who supports and enables an alcoholic or drug addict. But it can also refer to someone who's unable to cope with life without having another person around, whether there are drugs involved or not. It's the "I can't live without you" syndrome, and can be related to having a separation anxiety disorder as a child as a result of suffering some sort of a loss, or it can simply be related to poor parenting.

Codependent people place their own needs beneath those of others and are consumed with making others happy. Ironically, codependent people are attracted to narcissists because narcissists place their own needs above everyone else's, and they rely on codependent people to clean up all their messes. Codependent people, on the other hand, are constantly looking for someone else's mess to clean up. A codependent and a narcissist are a match made in heaven, or hell.

Some of the few things I still have from when I was a child are report cards from my early school years. In every one of them there are check marks reprimanding me for not respecting other people's property, having bad boundaries, and not keeping to myself, all red flags for codependency. As I got older, my codependency continued to grow unabated until it spread into every relationship I've ever had with another human being. Finally, one day a recovering alcoholic friend of mine told me I was codependent, but I had never even heard the word before, and I had no idea what it meant. It wasn't until I started going to therapy that I really started to understand. My therapist also told me I was codependent, and when I asked her what that meant she said, "It's not knowing where you end and where someone else begins," and something about bad boundaries. That sounded profound but I thought, "what the hell is that supposed to mean?" So I got rid of my therapist and began my journey of trying to figure it out on my own.

At that point, I had learned that one of the core features of being codependent was having bad boundaries, but I still didn't understand what that meant. I guess it was the word "boundaries" that was throwing me off. I knew what the word meant literally, I played sports my whole life, but I was having trouble applying it figuratively, or behaviorally. Then I learned that limit-setting is how children are first taught about having boundaries. This led me to the best definition I could find: boundaries are physical or psychological lines that should not be crossed by you or by anyone else. Boundaries maintain order in relationships, and without them there is always chaos and drama. Now, the concept seemed so simple to understand, but I couldn't believe no one told me this in the first place, like when I was a child, and I can only imagine the difference it would have made.

Having bad boundaries involves over-the-line behavior, like when someone takes something they know isn't theirs, or when someone touches someone else without their permission; these are examples of having bad physical boundaries. Bad psychological boundaries are when people provide too much personal information too soon in a relationship, or when you tell someone you love them on the first date. It's the teenager who's spending too much time with their new love and neglecting their own priorities like schoolwork or spending time with their own family. Perhaps a codependent teenager's target is their peer group, where the teenager's whole life revolves around socializing with the peer group and all other aspects of their life start to fall apart; then drugs and alcohol get involved and the rest is history. Having bad boundaries means that you allow your own time or space to be invaded by others, even though you're getting hurt in the process. Some of these people love to play the victim role and are constantly dramatizing about how everyone in their life has taken advantage of them in some way, when all they had to do was say "no". You may think that you already understand all of this, but I'll bet you that without knowing it, you regularly let other people invade your own boundaries, or you often cross the line into other people's territory without permission.

Learning about all of this boundary stuff has made me realize how, not only is a large part of our society narcissistic, but there's also an equally large part that is very codependent. This makes sense because one group cannot live without the other. The narcissistic part of society is constantly trying to invade everyone's Self with drama, sales pitches, advertisements and bad ideas - trying to get people to sacrifice their time, money, or attention. The weakest codependent stragglers at the back of the herd end up getting consumed by this narcissistic black hole of drama and sensory overload. The way things are now makes it even more important to understand that boundaries are the glue that holds our society, as well as our Self, together; without them we just fall apart. Without educating ourselves about boundaries, the lines that separate everything and everyone will be blurred.

Once this picture of codependence became clearer to me, I began to see that I had spent a good bit of my life being codependent, especially in my close relationships. When I was dating someone, I would always put myself last, and my entire world revolved around making them happy. I would think they were the most amazing person in the world, and that I didn't deserve to be with them because they were so amazing and I wasn't. This would go on for a while until I was completely drained. Then my projections of them being god-like would disappear and I'd drop them like a hot potato. I would finally start to feel good again, gaining just enough confidence to meet someone else, and do it all over again; it was exhausting.

Some people are much more codependent than others, which means that they just have to work harder than everyone else to be whole. Many people will also never be able to figure out the deep Freudian causes of their dysfunctions, and that's ok because this is usually not necessary in order for them to improve their behavior. I, however, was determined to understand the reason why I was so screwed up. It seemed like such a mystery that I just had to solve, and it took me years of research and self-examination, but I think I finally figured it out. I also wanted to do everything I could to prevent my daughter from having to go through the emotional slaughter that I did. Now keep in mind that there are many different causes to people's dysfunctions. For myself, however, I determined that the root cause of my own dysfunctions was due to the fact that my parents were struggling with their own mental demons and barely keeping it together themselves. The chaos of their struggle left little room for caring for me, and this left me out in the emotional cold.

I know what you're thinking, "She's blaming everything on her parents". But this discussion is not about placing blame, it's about learning why our thinking and behavior is less than ideal, so that we can think and behave better in the future. It's also about learning from our mistakes, and the mistakes of our parents, so that we are not destined to repeat them in the upbringing of our own children.

Now, I must tell you that what I went through might not be that impressive, and to those who need blood and guts and all that, I apologize. Nobody died here, I didn't have my leg bit off by a shark, I wasn't locked in a closet for thirteen years, and you probably won't see me on Oprah telling my story, but this really messed me up, and I think there are a lot of people out there who have underestimated the impact their upbringing has had on their own behavior.

I've already mentioned that my mother had a "nervous breakdown", which is what she always referred to it as, when I was about six years old. One time, I asked her if she remembered what happened, and she said she was trying to put my father in the hospital for his rage disorder, and the next thing she knew, they strapped her down and put her in the hospital. I'll never know for sure exactly what happened, but what I am sure of is that when it did happen, my whole world shattered into a million pieces. My mother mysteriously disappeared one day and I had no idea what was happening. All I remember was my dad saying that she was in the hospital and that she would be gone for a while; then he started crying. I have never before or since heard a grown man cry, and I will never forget that sound for as long as I live.

My mother ended up being in the hospital for what seemed like several months. The only other thing I remember was going to the hospital so my dad could see her, but my brother and I weren't allowed to visit her, I guess because she was so *bad off*. Perhaps my aversion to hospitals stems from this period in my life. Anyway, my brother and I would play downstairs in the hospital lobby with empty pill bottles and medicine cups until my dad came back acting like everything was fine. The next thing I remember was the day my mother finally came back home; she was highly medicated and seemed like a totally different person. I spent the rest of my childhood trying to make my tranquilized yet still depressed mother happy, while at the same time trying to deal with what turned into a profound separation anxiety disorder within myself. My childhood was filled with fear and confusion, and I often had no idea what to do with myself because my parents never talked to me about anything important.

The underlying psychology of how codependence and separation anxiety can develop is quite fascinating. Sometime around Kindergarten, children need to start emotionally separating from their parents. Apparently, if this separation process doesn't take place properly, you're screwed. I remember when my mom took me to my first day of kindergarten, I felt like she was throwing my blood-soaked body into shark-infested waters; I was convinced I would die that day. My kindergarten teacher had to tear me away from my mother, kicking and screaming bloody murder. I remember all the other kids were just calmly sitting down, watching me with their mouths wide open, but it didn't matter, I WAS GOING TO DIE! From that point on, I was terrified of going to school or going anywhere without my mother for the rest of my childhood. To this day, I often feel anxious leaving my family at home while I go out into the world.

In order for the separation process to take place properly, a parent needs to create a healthy connection to their child by fulfilling their emotional needs for love and attention. This isn't hard to accomplish if the parent has their own Self together. All they have to do is love and challenge the child, provide consistency and structure, make them feel visible, build their confidence, and make them feel safe. They can try to avoid confusing them with mixed messages, and mentally prepare them for what to expect in life. The separation process can then take place, with the parents carefully nudging the chicks out of the nest, letting them know that they can do it, and telling the children that they will be there to catch them if they fall.

The sad truth is that many children fail to make it through this separation process successfully. If the parents are miserable themselves, they usually are unable to meet their child's basic emotional needs for love and attention. These parents are constantly ignoring the child, snapping at them, or just pushing them away. The child interprets this as rejection, and they blame themselves for this. This is one of the few times in their lives when it would be totally acceptable to blame their parents for their problems, but most children will take full responsibility for it. The reason they do this is because it would be too frightening for a small child to think that the reason her parents are not taking care of her properly and making her feel loved is because her parents have no idea what they're doing, so she instead blames herself. Now the child believes that her parents' unhappiness is her fault, and that she doesn't *deserve* their love. So to fix the problem, she sets out to try to be *better* to make her parents happy, which of course is an impossible task. Having never made it through the separation process successfully, these children will grow up seeking out emotionally unavailable partners, trying to recreate the relationship with their dysfunctional parents so they can somehow make everything right. The problem is that this doesn't work, and they will continue to fail to make other people happy until, hopefully one day, they realize that the only person they really need to make happy is themselves.

My mother struggled with the chaos in her mind her entire life, and while the weight of her psychological burdens was almost too much for her to bear, I know in her heart she believes she did the best she could as a parent. Unfortunately though, I needed so much more. Her drama and struggle got most of her attention, so there was little left to give to me. I've spent my entire life trying to fill the void that was left in her wake.

*

Once the codependent stage of life is set, many people never figure out what their problem is, and spend the rest of their life making the same mistakes, over and over again. The fortunate ones will figure it out, but only after years of pain and failed relationships. We must understand that the door to peace is in our hearts and minds, and that the best way through it is by building up our low self-esteem through reparenting ourselves. When I say reparenting, I'm talking about taking care of ourselves now as an adult, the way we wish we would have been taken care of as a child. We have to tell ourselves that we will be the ones to catch ourselves when we fall because no one else will, and that the opportunity to connect with our parents is probably long gone, and that we must reconnect with ourselves instead. We have to be willing to look at ourselves in the mirror and say to ourselves the things that we wish we could have heard from our parents. We have to tell ourselves that it's okay to not be perfect because as the old saying goes, "the only perfect people are in the graveyard". We have to tell ourselves that we know how we feel because life is sometimes quite challenging, and we have to tell ourselves that we can accomplish difficult things because "if someone can do it... anyone can do it."

Chapter 16

PARENTING

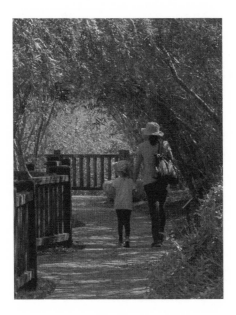

Once we have reparented ourselves, repaired all of the damage done to us from our childhood, and relocated our family away from the hazardous waste dumps, we can then provide our own children with the upbringing we wish we would have had. I was never sure about being a parent because I never thought I would be any good at it. Besides, I was hardly giving my plants and animals enough love and attention. It also seemed like so much work, and I was busy doing so many very important things (NOT!). So that's why it was such a surprise that when I finally did become a parent, I felt like my daughter was the most important person in the world to me, and I couldn't imagine my life without her. When she was born, it suddenly became my purpose in life to make sure she had all the mental tools that I never had. But I didn't feel like I had a knack for parenting, and I was afraid that I would do or say something stupid that would traumatize her for the rest of her life. So I made sure that I not only studied all the things I should do, I also learned all the things that I shouldn't do.

Besides beating your children, smoking cigarettes around them and letting them watch TV all the time are probably at the top of the list of "things not to do". I'm pretty sure that my mother was smoking a cigarette at the moment that she gave birth to me to calm her down, and transcripts of Tom and Jerry are emblazoned on my brain from the countless hours I spent watching it. So while I spent my childhood watching Tom and Jerry cartoons and Gilligan's Island reruns, over and over, for what seemed liked years in our claustrophobic house, my parents chain-smoked in silence with all the windows shut. Every other day, my mother would interrupt my TV shows to send me to the White Hen Pantry to buy her two packs of cigarettes for fifty cents, with a note scribbled on a torn-up piece of paper that said, "Please give my daughter 2 packs of Virginia Slims menthol, Thank You," and she would officially date and sign it. Even more astonishing is that the store clerk actually sold me the cigarettes.

My mother decided at an early age that nothing she ever did made much of a difference in life, so why bother trying; it just wasn't worth the effort. In my mother's defense, she didn't have the best upbringing herself, and she had some major psychological battles to fight, battles that she could never seem to win. Fortunately, the only thing my mother ever really passionately wanted to do was to have children; such is the power of the biological urge, it can overcome even hopeless depression. Her unhappiness and feelings of being helpless to improve the quality of her life returned sometime after the shine of giving birth wore off. This was when the "learned helplessness" of my mother started to rub off on me. As a result, it took me decades to realize that I was the one who had all the control in my life, not everyone and everything else.

"Learned helplessness" was first theorized by Martin Seligman, a professor of psychology at the University of Pennsylvania, and is based on experiments related to depression that he conducted at the university starting in 1967. What he and his fellow researchers found was that when animals were exposed to adverse situations that they could not avoid, they learned to behave helplessly. The next time they were in a similar situation, except that this time they were given a chance to escape, they would not leave their unpleasant circumstance, even though the door was wide open. Seligman compared this behavior to that of humans who are severely depressed and often perceive an absence of control over their lives.

In one study, dogs were repeatedly exposed to electric shocks that they could not escape from. Ultimately, the dogs stopped trying to escape the shocks, even if an opportunity to escape was presented to them; they *learned* to behave as if they were helpless. People who are depressed often believe that they cannot escape the unpleasant aspects of their lives because they have failed to do so in the past, so they give up trying. To help them cope with the discomfort, their threshold for pain becomes elevated and they just get used to it.

Another experiment was done with people who performed mental tasks in the presence of a distracting noise. People who had no control over the noise did poorly, while those who could use a switch to turn off the noise did much better, even though they rarely used the switch. Just knowing that they had the option to use the switch to turn off the noise diminished the distraction. Such is the power of being aware of your options and knowing how much control you really have.

To avoid being sucked into the black hole of *learned helplessness*, children need to be taught that they have some control over their environment, and this process needs to take place from the moment they are born. When they cry, they need to be picked up and soothed. When they're being cute, they need to be smiled at, and when they start to speak, they need to be spoken back to. Thus, one of the best things we can do as parents is make our children feel seen and heard; we need to make them feel visible by responding to their basic needs. As we have discussed in the relationship section, providing psychological visibility to another person is one of the greatest gifts we can give them, and it is crucial to raising a confident and well-adjusted child.

When they're old enough to start troubleshooting things, helping children learn how to fix their own problems is equally as important, instead of fixing everything for them. I'm not talking about abandoning them and letting them fend for themselves in a sea of sharks, I'm talking about leading them to their own solutions. This is challenging for parents initially because it can be time-consuming. It's a lot easier and faster to just fix their problems for them, but the damage caused by these bad parental habits will result in a lifetime of them playing victim because they never learn how to fix their own problems. Dr. Laura Markham of ahaparenting.com tells us that by taking this extra time with our child, they will build new brain pathways to talk themselves through challenging situations in the future. Taking this extra time with children early on will pay off in spades, as their newfound independence will feed on itself and will ultimately create more time for parents in the future.

*

Another pitfall of poor parenting is talking down to your children, rather than speaking to them as if they're adults. Of course there's exceptions to this, as you are the parent and at times need to be disciplinary. But as a general rule, children hate being spoken down to, and crave being treated as "big girls" or "big boys", with as much respect and dignity as adults get. Again, when they fall and scrape their knee, you should definitely soothe them. Hell, even at my age, if I hurt myself and I don't get a little sympathy, I still feel like crying. But when I hear someone speaking to their eight-year-old like they're four, using simple words and simple sentences, I cringe. The irony here is that these are the same parents that complain about how their children act so immature. If you treat your kid like a child, they'll act like one.

At the other end of the extreme is teaching your children that they have all the control. I've lost count how many times I've heard parents say, "They won't listen to me," when talking about their kids, or "I could never get them to do that!". We live in Southern California and the sun is blinding, literally, so we've been putting sunglasses on our daughter from birth. Of course she didn't want to wear them at first, and often took them off, but once she learned that this was the way it was gonna be, she left them on and now wears them all the time without a problem. People were always shocked at seeing a six-month-old wearing sun glasses, it was like she was in the circus or something. They would always say, "How do you get her to keep them on, my child rips them off and breaks them every time I try to put them on." So the question here is a simple one, "Who's the boss?" Oftentimes, it's the child.

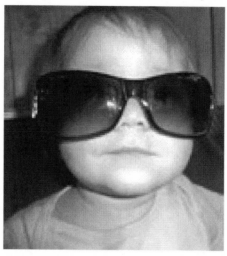

When my partner and I decided to have a child, we had no idea what we were doing, and we knew it. So we read several child-rearing books and taught ourselves the ropes, which apparently, most people don't do. Now, it's fascinating watching how other people raise their kids. "Sammy, stop throwing sand! Or why don't you just throw it at the tree, that's ok." Sammy's confused now, "Is throwing sand ok or not?", he thinks to himself. Well, two-year-old logic dictates that if throwing sand at a tree is ok, throwing sand must always be ok, and besides, Sammy's getting more attention from throwing sand than he's had all day, so Sammy now decides that throwing sand is great and he should do it all the time. This is the dead-end result of mixed messages, which many kids get throughout their childhood, so they end up basing all of their important decisions in life on faulty logic. "Don't do that!", you tell them, but they do it anyway and then you give up trying to discipline them because you suck at it. Now the child realizes that they have total control because you decided that you don't have any, and the rest is history. Limit-setting with children is like wearing a seat belt, you have to do it all the time or it doesn't work. Calm, consistent discipline is key.

Children crave a certain degree of structure and discipline in their lives, and when they don't get it, they act out. Time-outs are life savers for parents and children.

Another priceless virtue to teach your child is delayed-gratification. Research on this subject was conducted by Walter Mischel and his infamous "Marshmallow Test". Four-year-olds were placed in a room at a table with a marshmallow on it. They were told that they could either eat that marshmallow now, or if they waited to eat it for a little while, they could then have two marshmallows. Watching the children taking part in this study is fascinating and hilarious at the same time, but what Mischel found when he followed up with these kids some forty years later was that the group that waited for two marshmallows was more successful in several life measures, such as school performance, career success, and overall health. The key to take away here is that each time your child delays gratification, they build stronger brain pathways associated with self-discipline. So helping your child realize opportunities to "profit" from delayed gratification will be another powerful tool for them to add to their mental toolbox.

*

A few more tips that I picked up along the way:

-Besides teaching your child how to learn from their mistakes, getting them to recognize, value, and think about their accomplishments will do wonders for their self-esteem. This should be an event that takes place regularly throughout one's life.

-Learning to play a musical instrument does more for a child's brain than almost anything else.

-Children who develop an affinity and appreciation for books are considerably more successful than those who don't.

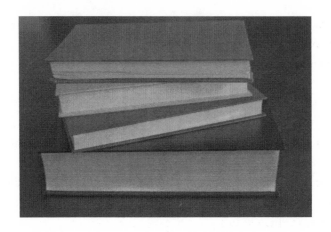

For the life of me, I cannot remember either one of my parents ever reading me a book. I do remember the Hefty bags full of Harlequin Romance books that my mother read herself through each week after her soap operas were over. On the rare occasions when I did have my face in a book, I would just look at the pictures because actually reading the book seemed like so much extra work, so I never did it unless I was forced to, and then I hated it. So I swore to myself that our daughter would love books. We started reading her books in utero, and by the age of two and a half, she was memorizing books cover to cover and reciting them to her stuffed animals that were gathered in a semi-circle in front of her. She's been to the library once a week, every week, for the last five years, and she still loves going there. She's read and memorized almost every book in the children's section and can show you exactly where many of them are on the shelf, so I can only imagine how large the repertoire of helpful information in her brain is, and I can only imagine how helpful this would have been for me and my life if I learned to love books as a child. So turn the TV off and take your kids to the library. Besides, most of the book stores are going bankrupt now and it could be you and your child's last chance to see a building full of books. For the record, our child gets about an hour of educational TV time a couple times a week while we cook dinner, but that's after spending all day with her, reading, teaching, and exploring life with her. She can also trade TV time for computer time if the games she plays are educational.

*

I've already told you how inspiring my parents were when I was growing up. I vividly remember how they would both be chain smoking in the car with the windows rolled up on the way to dropping me off at kindergarten. When I climbed out of the car, there would be an ominous cloud of grey smoke emanating off my coat that followed me into school. I always smelled like a dirty ashtray, and it's a wonder I'm still alive now. I thought that watching them blow smoke out of their mouths was the coolest thing in the world. I would always buy those fake candy cigarettes from the little store on the corner with my allowance; my parents thought it was so cute, a chip off the old block! They still sell those candy cigarettes by the way, I had to tell my five-year-old daughter she couldn't have them just the other day; so much for federal oversight. Maybe they should start selling candy crack pipes too, that would be cool, "Look Mom, I'm smoking crack! Just kidding."

The best thing my mother did for me was make me go to church, but that didn't save me though, I thought the kids from church were boring. Then one day, a bus pulled up in front of my grammar school. It was full of the bad kids from the bad school that had just closed down. I thought those bad kids were the coolest people I'd even seen in my life, so I decided to become one of them; why not, right? It was all downhill from there.

One of the first things I started teaching my daughter was all about the bad boys and girls, how they dress, where they hang out, the bad things they do, how they hurt people, and how they can hurt her. It's fascinating seeing the wheels turn in her mind when we talk about these things. I realize I'm running the risk of making the bad people seem appealing, so I'm very careful when I talk about them. If she does decide to hang out with them though, at least her decision will be an informed one, as opposed to how I had no idea what I was getting myself into. I want her to know all about them so when they try to seduce her with their fake charm, maybe she'll know better. I spend even more time pointing out what healthy, cool people look like... they look like me! I never knew how to spot the cool healthy people, and because they're usually quieter than the loud, obnoxious bad people, I never really noticed them. I was always attracted to the "life of the party people" who had multiple personality disorders. So to prepare my daughter, I

172

go as far as I can to explain things, but more importantly, I ask her what she thinks about it all, because I can't read her mind and I want to know if I'm on the right track. We give her choices about everything and let her make as many decisions about her life as is reasonable. We also make her feel visible, and she knows that everything she does is important to the whole family. Hopefully, this will help guide her into an amazing and pleasurable time as a teenager, rather than the confusing, depressing, and slaughterous teenage years that I went through.

*

As a poorly educated, rebellious teenager with bad boundaries and emotionally unavailable parents, I got kicked out of the house and was homeless by the time I reached eighteen. Once I realized that living in my car for the rest of my life was an unsustainable path, I tried to figure out what to do with my life. With absolutely no direction from my parents, I had no idea; I didn't even know what I was good at. At wits end, I considered enlisting in the military; it seemed like my only hope. I think this is what many lost teenagers consider, but it's not a bad gig if you think about it. The military provides great benefits such as education, discipline and structure; all of the things many of these kids never had. There are also many smart, high-performing teens that consider the military as a life's dream or career path, but the military has surely saved many lost souls and turned many hopeless lives around. I went so far as to talk to a recruiter and watch the introduction video. I knew I could get into the military if I wanted to, but all of the structure and discipline must have scared me because I chickened out at the last minute. This was probably a blessing in disguise because God knows what I would have done with a gun in my hand.

I had always been under the impression that anyone could get into the military if they really wanted to. Someone that I used to know, who was a total loser, got into the military, so I figured if he could get in, anyone could get in. Apparently though, that's not the case. According to the Department of Defense, approximately 71% of the 34 million 17 to 24-year-olds in this country would be rejected from the military if they tried to enlist, due to physical, behavioral, or educational shortcomings. In other words, the vast majority of young adults in our country are not qualified to serve in our armed forces. This is frightening from a defense standpoint, but what about the millions of lost and rejected teens who try to get into the military and potentially have their lives turned around? Most of them are now being rejected because they can't even qualify to do that; what are they going to do now? Once you get rejected from the military, there are not a lot of options left. A generation or two ago, they probably would have been accepted into the military, but now they're not thin enough, they're not healthy enough, and they're not smart enough. This is a low point in our country's history, and a clear reflection of how poor parenting is becoming a national crisis. It's time for us to step up our parenting game by building a stronger foundation for our children to build their lives upon so they can be fit for any kind of life they choose.

*Some other helpful parenting hints:

*teach your child early how to love being alone.

*Praise your child's strengths instead of criticizing their weaknesses; this will help build a strong foundation of trust, support, and good feelings at home which will make it easier for them to resist negative peer pressure.

*Disapprove of the behavior, not the child. They must know that you still love them, even though you disapprove of their behavior, or they will value their peer's acceptance and comfort over yours, which makes peer pressure way more powerful.

*Being a successful parent requires continuously monitoring our own behavior and approaches to our children, and reminding ourselves that their behavior is quite often a reflection of our own.

I haven't had the pleasure of experiencing my daughter's teenage years yet, and I remain cautiously optimistic because I know all too well the dangers that lie ahead. But I also know that if I prepare her well, her teenage years will be some of the best in her life.

Chapter 17

WORK

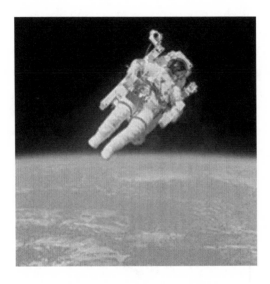

"As a day well spent procures a happy sleep, so a life well employed procures a happy death." - Leonardo Da Vinci

Most people don't like their jobs. According to an article in the Washington Post, a recent Gallup poll found that only thirteen percent of employees worldwide really like their jobs. I can think of many unpleasant jobs out there, like being a coal miner, or the people who have to clean up murder scenes. The other day I saw one of my neighbor's work trucks outside their house that was advertising "Around-The-Clock Live Killer Bee's Nest Removal"; that would suck too. I'm grateful that I don't have to do those jobs, although sometimes it feels like a swarm of bees is landing on me when I walk in the door of the Intensive Care Unit. People are screaming, alarms are going off, people are dying, there's not enough help, ugh!!! Why am I still doing it after twenty years? Well, I'm good at it, I love saving people's lives, and I have a lot of vacation time. Don't get me wrong, nurses are amazing and the job we do is extremely important, but the rising costs of healthcare and the cuts being made are making it very challenging to actually enjoy the job.

I finally realized, after I had been going to the same job with a knot in my stomach for twenty years, that it wasn't going to get any better; and I was destined to feel this way for the rest of my life. I began feeling a sense of urgency about trying to do something different. I kept hearing that little voice in the back of my head questioning if I was ever going to make my move out of there, and that if I didn't do it soon it would be too late. I knew that the only thing I would regret on my deathbed was not at least trying to do something different, something that gave me butterflies in my stomach, instead of knots.

An effective bandage for disliking your job is to lower your expectations, and in some cases, raise your threshold for pain. But these should be only temporary remedies because if used long-term, they could create a lifetime of having your job be your greatest source of unhappiness. Unfortunately, this is the plight of many. It is possible though, for your job to be one of your greatest sources of joy. If your purpose in life can somehow be incorporated into your job, then you will be driven by the fuel that is injected into your soul from doing what you love to do, and you could go on this way forever, loving life, and finding magic in each moment of your existence.

The "Life Deferral" Plan

I am so thankful for everything that I have in my life, and there's just one other thing that would make my life complete: if I could do something that I love and get paid for it. I don't know anyone who loves their job, most people say "it's ok" when you ask them about it. But oh how I crave to be one of those people who lives, eats, and breathes their job. I know it's possible because every now and then I read about someone who has a dream job. In fact, just the other day I was reading an article in Oprah Magazine about Dolly Parton who's been in the music business for over 52 years. Dolly was talking about how much she loves her job, and she said in her cute little country voice, "I hope to fall over dead on stage right in the middle of a song". That's how I want to feel about my job. I want to love it so much that I want to die while I'm doing it. Instead, I feel like my job is killing me. Dolly Parton also sings one of my favorite songs,"9 to 5", and at one point in the song Dolly sings in her cute little country voice, "There's a better life, and you think about it don't you?"; and every time I hear that song, I think about it.

I finally decided to pursue "a better life" when I read one of the most inspiring books ever, *The 4-Hour Workweek*, by Timothy Ferriss. This book changed the course of my life forever. I knew I had to do something different, and reading this book alone gave me more inspiration than anything else. Timothy Ferriss explains that most people are on what he calls the "life deferral" plan, which he describes as struggling most of your life at jobs you don't enjoy, trying to save enough money to hopefully someday retire, if you live that long and survive the struggle. He colorfully describes how "the math doesn't work" and that in the end you'll be screwed because you sold yourself short waiting for "someday". Reading this book forced me to admit that this was how I was living my life. I realized that I couldn't go on this way any longer, so I started formulating a solid plan to get the hell out of Dodge.

The first thing I had to do was figure out exactly what I wanted to do with my life. One of my favorite lines is from one of the first and best self-help books that I ever read, *Life Strategies* by Phil McGraw: "You have to name it to claim it." It's also one of the first lines I taught my two-year-old daughter. What I learned from this book is that no one ever teaches us how to figure out what we want to do with our lives. We all take for granted that our brains will magically lead us in the right direction. We have been taught our whole lives to recognize what we don't want; we're really good at that, after all, we've been complaining about what we don't want for decades. The hard part is figuring out what we do want, and many of us have never even taken the time to consider it because we've been too busy complaining. No one ever asks us what we want either, usually because most people don't care what we want. If you want to shut someone up who is endlessly complaining, try asking them what they want, and they'll usually be speechless. We have to be able to spell out in fine detail what it is we want. You can go around in circles for the rest of your life, but until this happens, nothing else will.

So I sat down and looked at my life, and for the first time, I made a list of all the things I love to do the most. I was determined to create a situation where I woke up every morning eager to start my day, and not just on my days off. I had to keep reminding myself that the only person who could stop me was myself with my negative thinking. I had to become my own defensive paratrooper and constantly shoot down and counterattack each reason that I (or anyone else for that matter) came up with as to why my plan wouldn't work, and you know what? It actually worked. I was surprised at how many more reasons I came up with to defend and support what I was doing.

After I made my list of the three or four things that I love to do the most, I started weaving them together into something that I could potentially pay the bills with. I love going to hardware stores, I love building stuff, I loved writing in college and I was pretty good at it, I've been studying psychology my entire life, and God knows I've read enough self-help books. So I built myself a studio in my backyard, and now I'm writing this book. If no one buys it, then I'll write a children's book because God knows I've read enough of those. If no one buys that, then I'll carve cherubs out of tree trunks and sell them out of my garage or something... I don't know. All I know is that I'm having more fun than I ever had in my life. I just keep reminding myself that the more I love what I do, the more beautiful and valuable what I do will be.

The next thing I did was to significantly cut down my hours at work. I knew immediately that this was the right decision because I couldn't remember the last time I was so excited about anything. Even though I'd be living check to check and it was significantly decreasing my financial security, it didn't matter. It felt like I had a new lease on life, and I had butterflies in my stomach. I never knew how much fun life could be. It's kind of like never really being in love with someone, you just don't know how it feels until it really happens.

Keep in mind, there are rules that apply to this strategy, like the bills have to be paid on time and the children have to go to school, etc. You have to be prepared and you have to have a plan that passes muster with the spouse and kids. Once you get everyone on board and the stage is set for your debut, it can be a little daunting because now you have to perform what you've been talking about for so long, that thing that you've been dying to do. This is the moment of truth because if you've put everything together well in your head, then you'll be so excited about what you're doing that you'll just do it. If not, you'll stumble out of the gate and have to reevaluate everything. Being able to visualized your plan beforehand is an effective tool because then when you implement it - it's like you've already done it to some extent, and it will be more likely to work.

Of course, money is always an issue, and some people will have to work a lot harder and be more financially creative than others to make this work, and that's just the way it is. If you want it bad enough though, you can make it happen. When I cut my hours at work, something happened that I didn't expect. My pre-planned budget indicated that we would essentially be living check-to-check until I figured out how to make some more money. I had been working on this budget for about a year before I put my plan into effect, so I thought I had cut everything down to the bone. Once I went part-time though, ironically, we were still saving some money. It turned out that being happier all the time made it even easier to save money. When I was working so hard at my unpleasant and thankless job, I felt like I was entitled to buy more stuff to make up for the discomfort of my job; it was like I had to fill the void with the stuff. Now the void was smaller, so I didn't need as much stuff. I also didn't need to drink as much alcohol to ease the pain, and we didn't go out to eat as much because staying at home and cooking with the family was more enjoyable. So the money is there, you just have to do a little searching. Merely starting the process of observing the situation makes things that you had no idea were there... suddenly appear. If you never bother to look, you won't find it.

*

Many people spend their lives driving down the highway of life looking in the rearview mirror, not even realizing that they're headed in the wrong direction, or that perhaps they missed their exit. When I was on the *life deferral* plan, the vision I had of my life was foggy at best. What I could see was that I would probably be working at the same job for the rest of my life, and that was okay... it was a good job, but it made me sad. When I drove past the cemetery on the way to work every day, it was like the spirits were talking to me and mocking me from their graves, "What are you gonna do girlfriend? Are you gonna wait a little longer... there's always more time, right? Ha, ha, ha!" Oh, the conversations I've had in my head driving past that cemetery. They're different now though, and I don't drive past it as often, but when I do, it's almost as if the spirits are cheering me on now.

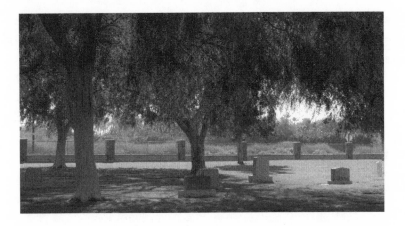

I forgot to mention one more benefit of the new path you've chosen to take in life: your brain's going to love what you're doing, because doing something new and exciting with your life builds new brain pathways. Nothing makes the brain shrink more than doing the same old thing, in the same place, over and over again.

Chapter 18

BRAIN

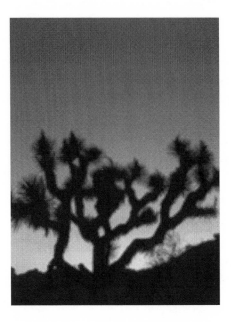

By now, you're well on your way to mastering your mind, and while you're at it, it will be motivating to remind yourself that you're physically changing your brain and creating new brain pathways with each moment you spend on trying to improve yourself. We've already talked a little about brain plasticity, but I must emphasize that the more aware you are of this phenomenon, of how each thought that enters your mind changes your brain and can transform your life, the more motivated you will be to have positive thoughts.

Brain plasticity simply means that the brain is constantly transforming itself. If you don't use your brain and instead keep doing the same things all of the time, brain cells die and unused pathways disappear. If you are continuously learning and challenging yourself, the birth of new brain cells and the creation of new brain pathways can occur throughout one's life.

Unfortunately, it wasn't until recently that scientists started taking the possibility of brain plasticity seriously. It had been generally accepted that once a part of the brain died, the function that part of the brain served could no longer be recovered. The most amazing and inspiring book ever written on this subject is *The Brain That Changes Itself,* by Norman Doidge, who discusses how the scientific community finally figured out that, even after part of the brain has died, it can "reorganize" itself so that the good part of the brain takes over for the part that has died. If you had a stroke in the past, your fate was sealed. Now we know that it's possible, in many cases and with intensive therapy, to get back a significant part of the function that was lost, but only if you're rich and famous, and have really good health insurance, or if you have a big family that's willing to do all the physical therapy for free.

Scientists have also figured out that one of the keys to maintaining brain plasticity is to keep our brains happy. If a dog is locked up in a yard all day, never getting exercise, never going anywhere new, never seeing and smelling new things, it will be angry, stressed, and miserable; it may even be foaming at the mouth. We're essentially causing similar damage to our brains by neglecting them in these ways.

Perhaps the best way to neglect our brains is to allow ourselves to be stressed out all the time. There's no question, based on the many studies that have been done, that stress and depression can kill brain cells by shrinking the gray matter in our brains and leading to learning, memory, and communication problems. But the damage can be repaired, and like intensive physical therapy can reverse the damage of a stroke, there are many things we can do to reverse the damage of a lifetime of stress, depression, and mediocrity.

One of the most powerful things we can do to increase brain plasticity is to exercise. It's amazing to me how few people actually do this consistently. According to the U.S. Bureau of Labor Statistics, only about sixteen percent of the population takes part in sports and exercise activities on an average day. There's also an interesting map at bls.gov that shows the distribution of which states in the U.S. exercise the most. If you live on the west coast, you're fifty percent more likely to exercise than if you're from most other parts of the country.

The brain also loves being in an enriched environment. When was the last time you surrounded yourself with something beautiful and just absorbed it, and maybe even got goose bumps from it? When was the last time you had a creative insight? When was the last time you got your heart rate up above its baseline for more than five minutes? Remember that little things can make a big difference. If you give your brain a little taste of something different and stimulating, it will pay you back in spades.

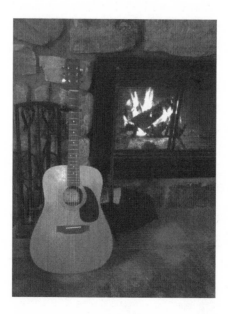

Most people's lives aren't all that mentally stimulating, so even if they aren't that stressed out, their brains are probably slowly shrinking from lack of use because they're on autopilot. They go to the same job that they already know how to do, they take the same route to work, and they dramatize about the same old stories with the same old people, and nothing ever really changes. Just doing something different, even if it's something small like using your left hand instead of your right, or walking backwards, can make a big difference to your brain; you have to mix things up a little in your life. Exercising, especially in new and different ways is at the top of the list of preventing your brain from shrinking. Learning a new language, playing a musical instrument, playing chess, learning how to juggle, martial arts, and even dancing should all be a part of your recipe for preserving and improving your brain.

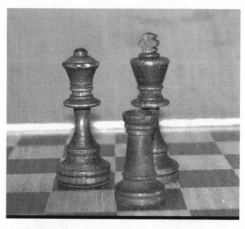

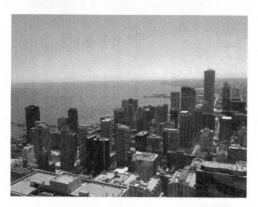

Simply looking at anything beautiful is very stimulating for the brain, so I've made it a point to surround myself with things that are visually appealing as much as possible. Chicago is one of the most beautiful cities in the world, but having spent most of my life there, I found I was always craving a more natural landscape, so I decided to move to southern California. Now, as I peer out of the window of my studio, instead of brick walls, I see one of the most beautiful mountainous landscapes in the world. Every time I step outside, I am in awe of the beauty that surrounds me. Chicago is beautiful in its own way, I love to visit it, and I even miss the brick walls sometimes. In my next house, I think I'll add a little brick wall in one of the rooms, but I wouldn't give up my beautiful scenery for anything now.

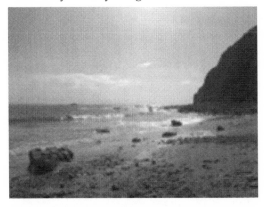

Knowing how powerful visually inspiring things are, I chose ten of the most beautiful and inspiring pictures I've ever seen and put them all over my studio, so that I'm surrounded by them all day long.

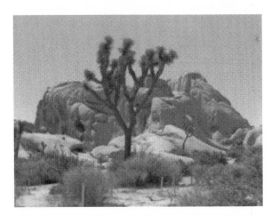

Chapter 19

VISION QUEST

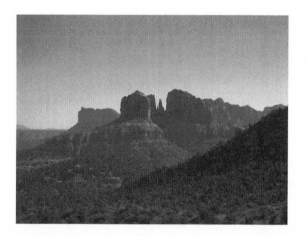

One of the most amazing tools of the mind, which can create new brain pathways and strengthen existing ones, is visualization. Using the mind to visualize anything you want is extremely powerful. It's so powerful that the most successful athletes, performers, and business people in the world use it to be at the top of their game. But I guess if you don't have a game, you don't really need to be on top of anything, so perhaps you could use visualization to figure out what your game should be.

Several studies, including research from the Cleveland Clinic, have shown that imagining you're exercising a muscle actually strengthens the muscle. Visualization gives us the ability to do just about anything in our minds, and this has saved the lives of countless prisoners of war and victims of concentration camps throughout history, yet most people aren't even aware that this power exists. So putting a little time and effort into practicing and perfecting this ability is well worthwhile.

Visualization is not that complicated, and the hardest part is merely taking the time to do it. Whatever it is that you want to do or practice doing, just close your eyes and imagine yourself doing it, step by step, in the greatest detail you can muster. Then, do it over and over again, each time with greater detail, stronger feelings, brighter colors, clearer sounds, clearer dialogue. It's as if you're creating, directing and editing a short film in your mind. The benefit comes from the fact that your brain has trouble telling the difference between imagining doing something and really doing it, so it's almost as if you're really doing it, and practice makes perfect.

I use visualization for everything, from giving a talk or having a conversation with someone, to building something big or even fixing something small. Perhaps, most importantly, I use it to see what I want my future to be like so that I can keep myself headed in the right direction.

Visualization can also help us learn from our mistakes without actually making them. In other words, we can evaluate the consequences of our actions by visualizing their impact before we really make our move.

*

Daydreaming is similar to visualization, except that unlike visualization, we're not always aware that we're doing it. Daydreams are usually thought of as pleasant, but for many people, they often contain negative mental imagery. A recent study conducted by the National Institutes of Health showed that people with anxiety disorders and/or major depression had a significantly greater ability to conjure up vivid negative imagery than those who didn't have these disorders. The study also showed that when anxious and depressed people were asked to deliberately generate positive imagery, their images were significantly less vivid than those without these disorders. So the bottom line is that you must realize when you're watching a horror movie in your mind, and change the channel to something more inspiring.

It's also important to understand the sequence of events that take place in your mind that lead to feelings of anxiety. First you have a negative thought, and if you don't stop the negative thought in its tracks, it will be followed by a negative visual image, which is then followed by you feeling like crap. At this point, you'll have one last chance to take control by challenging the negativity and trying to make yourself feel better before the whole day is ruined. If left unchecked, these toxic fantasies can wreak havoc in your mind, and remember, the brain has trouble telling the difference between fantasy and reality, so the damage to your body that the stress causes is almost as great as it would be if you really experienced the catastrophe. This is where visualizing a more positive scenario comes into play, and with practice you can turn the negative images into more positive ones.

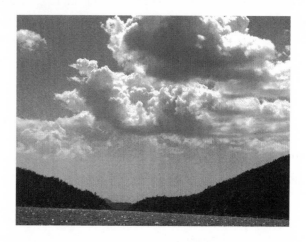

Vision boards are also powerful tools, and mine is filled with all the pictures that represent how I want my life to be. For years, I talked about making a vision board but never got around to it because it kept falling off my list. Finally, I made it a priority and put it together. Now, I can't believe how much I love looking at it because every time I do I automatically get a dose of endorphins. I put one on the wall next to my bed and I look at it every chance I get; I never get tired of looking at it. There are pictures of all of the most beautiful places I've been and want to revisit. There are pictures of my camper because that's how I want to visit those places, and my family because I don't want to go without them. I have pictures of my guitar, my studio, my telescope, and all the planets and galaxies I want to explore with it. When I made the board I realized that, for the first time, I was able to see all of things that I love the most in one place at the same time. I also realized that my 5-year-old daughter needed one too. She loves the ocean and everything in it, so she put an aquarium, a scuba diver and some fish on it for starters.

If you can't see whatever it is that you want in life, if you can't close your eyes and create that vision in your mind, then you probably haven't spent enough time trying to figure out what it is that makes you happy. I see things all the time in my mind, things that I want, different encounters with people, and I'm much more aware of my negative imagery. It's like there's a whole other world going on in my mind that I wasn't really aware of before. Now I am aware, and I'm learning how to harness and control these conscious or semi-conscious visions, but what about the unconscious visions, what about our dreams?

Chapter 20

DREAMS

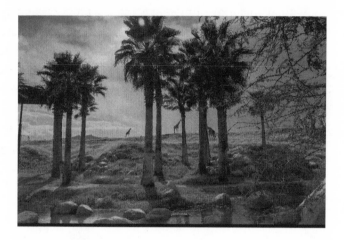

Sigmund Freud was one of the first people to describe dreams as being the doorway to our unconscious mind, and the more we remember and try to interpret our dreams, the more access we will have to the mind's infinite potential. Many believe that dreams are manifestations of our deepest hopes and fears. At the very least, they are messages from our unconscious about things that we have been preoccupied with during the day, and at the most they are the answers to life's most burning questions.

The fascination with dreams has been around since the beginning of time. Ancient Egyptians wrote down their dreams on papyrus, and those with vivid dreams were thought to be blessed, bringing messages from the gods. Dreams have also played a central role in many Native American tribes. They are used as a rite of passage and as guidance for the future. Perhaps even the cavemen and women were recording the visions in their dreams on the walls of the caves in France thirty thousand years ago.

Dreams can be pretty strange, and this may be related to the decreased activity in the prefrontal cortex, an area of our brain that is responsible for logic and planning. Dreams are believed to be an involuntary and unconscious phenomenon, where the person dreaming is completely unaware of what they are dreaming, and they are unable to control their behavior or anything else that happens within the dream. But there has also been some interesting research done suggesting the possibility of having conscious control of our dreams, called lucid dreaming. But whether we are conscious of our dreams or not, improving our ability to remember our dreams can be the first step in receiving the messages they may be sending. This can be challenging because most dreams are forgotten upon awakening. This may be due to the fact that the brain chemicals that convert short-term memories to long-term memories are suppressed during REM sleep. So keeping a dream journal is quite helpful for this, but it requires the discipline to write down the dream as soon as we wake up and before we do anything else.

*

It's amazing to me how many people are completely oblivious to what's going on in their minds while they sleep, where they spend about thirty percent of their entire lives. Sleeping and dreaming should be regarded as a powerful process before, during, and afterwards. Considering the questions of your life before you go to sleep can set up a dream stage whose purpose is to answer those questions, and writing your dreams down upon awakening will enhance this process.

For those of you who think that sleeping is an inconvenience and that the time allotted for sleep can be used more constructively, think again. This is perhaps the best example of "robbing Peter to pay Paul". If you're not getting enough sleep, you're taking years off your life, and diminishing the quality of your performance in many areas of your life in the process. For those of you who want to master your minds, it will very difficult to do without enough sleep.

191

According to research conducted by the National Institutes of Health, if the information we study and the things we learn are followed by a good sleep, this creates brand new memories and connections in the brain by replaying the information on a cellular level during sleep. I remember when I was in school, I took naps all the time while I was studying, and I was always at the top of my class. There have also been outrageous claims by some famous people in history, namely Edgar Cayce, the great American prophet, that by placing books next to their bed at night, they will have them memorized in the morning. Now you may never be able to perform this feat, but there's no denying the importance of sleeping and dreaming, and how not getting enough sleep impedes the learning process and destroys connections in our brain. I'm always surprised when I hear some people bragging about how little sleep they need, four or five hours a night for example. They must have done so much damage to their brains that they actually believe this is true.

Besides keeping us healthy, dreaming can also be linked to having creative breakthroughs. Many famous people have credited their success to a dream that ended up changing the world. August Kekule` saw the structure of benzene in a dream, and Albert Einstein had a dream that inspired his discovery of the key to the special theory of relativity, $E=mc2$. Now maybe you won't have an earth-shattering discovery like they did, but at the very least, you could uncover some hidden truths about your life in your dreams.

When I wake up in the morning and remember my dreams, it feels like I went to another place in time, another dimension. I'm always a little disappointed when I can't remember my dreams, but some people never remember their dreams at all. Many of these people think that they don't dream at all, but everybody dreams; it's just a matter of putting more effort into trying to remember them. Perhaps remembering the dreams we had while we were asleep will remind us of our life's dreams when we're awake. It's sad that some people often can't remember either.

*

Once we have converted the chaos in our minds back to order, pulled our Self back together, and created a detailed vision of our dreams, a tectonic shift begins to take place in our lives that can open the door to previously inaccessible powers of the mind. Many people are convinced that there is a definite limit to the power of the mind. Their narrow-mindedness stems from the fear of not knowing what they would do with such power if it did exist. But despite the criticism that surrounds the idea that our minds have infinite potential, there have been some mind-bending theories and discoveries that flirt with this possibility. These theories blend philosophy, physics, and biology together into a whole new dimension, making it harder than ever before for naysayers to simply dismiss the possibility of a limitless mind.

Chapter 21

MIND OVER MATTER

The Rolling Stones' song, *Ruby Tuesday*, has a great line in it, "...lose your dreams and you will lose your mind", and maybe that's just what happens to some people. But by having more control of our mind, maybe we will be better able to hold onto our dreams. We began in chapter one with "It's all in your head", meaning the path to our happiness or the path to our despair. It's horrible to think that things can get so bad for people that jumping off a bridge is the best solution they can come up with. The ultimate result of chaos in the mind is the desire to self-destruct, so we must share our knowledge of how to find peace and joy in an effort to get those who want to jump off a bridge to take a step back from the edge. Based on the statistics, there's a good chance that the life we save may be our own.

Things almost got that bad for me after I got kicked out of my house and had to live in my car for six months during a cold Chicago winter, with no friends, no family, and no future. It could have been much worse though, and lord knows how many people have had much more depressing experiences, but I never felt so alone in my life, and I thought about ending it all on a few occasions. Every time I did though, the one thing that stopped me was the fact that I didn't want to miss out on anything. I somehow knew that things would get better and I wanted to be there when they did. I will never forget how painful that time in my life was, and it still scares me to think of how close I came to the edge of oblivion. Unfortunately, for the 43,000 people that killed themselves this year, the pain of being alive was greater than the pain of missing out on life. Where exactly in their minds did they pass the point of no return, the point at which they were convinced that there would never be a better day? Is there also a corresponding point in our minds past which we'll never again have to return to the depths of despair and we'll know that, from now on, we'll be happier than we've ever been before? All I can say is that, for all those people who took their own lives, something went terribly wrong in their head when their mind told their body to destroy itself.

The Ghost In The Machine

The relationship between the mind and the body has been debated for the last several thousand years. On one side of the debate is the belief that the mind and body are two separate (dual) substances; this is called *dualism*, which states that the mind is non-physical and the brain is physical. Dualism suggests that the mind and thoughts are invisible *ghost-like* things, and that they are separate from the machine of your brain and body. This is where the phrase "the ghost in the machine" comes from, where the ghost is your mind and the machine is your physical body, including your brain.

This type of dualism, where the mind and body are separate substances, has come to be known as Cartesian dualism, named after the 17th century philosopher Rene Descartes. Dualism places much greater emphasis and value on the mind. Descartes believed, like Plato did, that enlightened people, such as those who climbed out of the cave in Plato's Allegory, should ignore the confused and shadowy messages from our physical senses and physical body, and instead focus on the bright world of the mind's clear and distinct thoughts and ideas.

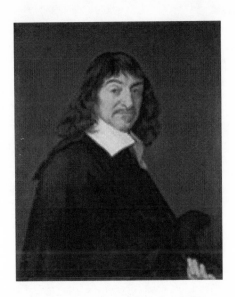

Monism, on the other hand and in contrast to dualism, argues that the mind and body are of one and the same substance; that is that they are both physical. Monists argue that their position is supported by findings in neuroscience which show that the creation and transmission of thoughts has been physically recorded with brain scans, proving that the thoughts of the mind are also physical and of the same substance as the body.

After hundreds of years of a general belief in dualism, believing that the brain is fixed and unchangeable, and that our thoughts are separate and have no lasting effect on the brain, a fascinating but tragic event became the first evidence in history to support monism and the theory that the mind and brain are both physical. It all started with a man named Phineas Gage (1823–1860) who, at the age of twenty-five, was working on the railroad packing explosive powder with a tamping rod. The powder unexpectedly exploded and sent the rod through his head. Phineas Gage miraculously survived the accident but the injury changed his personality, supposedly turning him into an angry drunk. Phineas Gage's mind seemed to be as damaged as his brain, so this was the first evidence to suggest that the mind and the brain are made of the same stuff. After losing his job at the railroad, Phineas Gage got a job driving coaches in Chile, and ended up dying at the age of thirty-six from seizures.

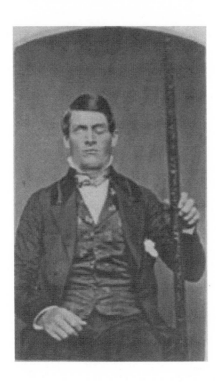

The term "the ghost in the machine" was originally coined by British philosopher Gilbert Ryle when he was discussing Descartes' dualism. *The Ghost In The Machine* is also a book that challenges the idea of dualism, written by Arthur Koestler, who also wrote *The Act of Creation* which I discussed in the chapter on creativity. The band *The Police* expressed their own views on dualism in 1981 with their most famous album, *The Ghost In The Machine*, with three top hits from it: "Every Little Thing She Does Is Magic", "Invisible Sun", and "Spirits in the Material World".

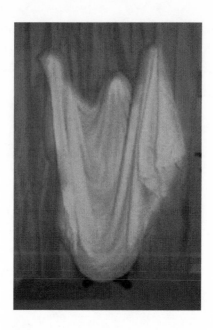

So what difference does it make whether or not the mind and body are one in the same? Well, do you believe in life after death? Some dualists believe that the mind and soul are immortal and live on once the body has died, while many monists believe that the mind dies with the body. Do you believe that the brain is fixed and unchangeable? Many dualists believe that our thoughts, being separate and mystical, have no real impact on our brain, making changing our brain with our minds impossible. What about free will? Do you believe your thoughts can change the course of your life? Some monists believe that the mind and body, being one in the same, are ruled by the classical laws of the universe. They believe these laws declare "free will" an illusion by stating that everything in our lives unfolds predictably before us based on mathematical equations, regardless of how we think. These beliefs have held back the positive psychology of the mind for the last century, and allowed many to believe that their lot in life was set, and that nothing they could do would change it. Fortunately, we are beginning to appreciate the astonishing power that the mind can have over the body, and that we really can change anything, if we put our minds to it.

So which is it, monism or dualism? Well, maybe it's both, but why does it matter? It matters because the dimension that allows monism and dualism to exist together is the same dimension that can give us a limitless mind. Only in this dimension can we have the safety and security of mainstream science, the beauty of an immortal soul, and the inspiration of free will, all at the same time. Our goal is to find the exact location of this place, and our journey will lead us not into the Twilight Zone, but to a place right next to it called quantum physics.

Let's Get Physical!

While the great philosophers of the last millennium have been battling over a definition of the relationship between the mind and body, a similar battle has been brewing over the last century between classical physicists and quantum physicists, specifically about how physics functions in the mind.

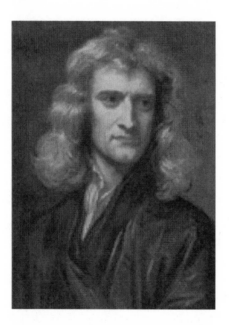

Physics is the study of the physical structure of stuff, it's shape and size, and how that stuff interacts with space and time. The roots of classical physics go back to the moment when Isaac Newton, pictured above, saw the apple fall from the tree. We're all familiar with gravity, Albert Einstein, and E=mc2, so we're all a little familiar with classical physics. Classical physics is the physics of big stuff, which is considered anything larger than an atom. One of the hallmarks of classical physics is that nothing can travel faster than the speed of light, or about 186,000 miles per second, which is the 'c' in E=mc2 (constant of light), and it plays a crucial role in Einstein's Special Theory of Relativity. Ironically, as amazing as classical physics and Einstein's theories are, some consider their contributions to the advancement of our species limited. The discovery of quantum physics, however, has shockingly transformed our understanding of the world as we know it. It has become the fuel that has powered great advances in many areas, especially technology, and we're just now beginning to realize the role it plays in the mind. It's impossible to understand the power of the mind without understanding quantum physics, but it will take a little work to wrap your mind around it.

$$E\psi = \frac{\hbar^2}{2m}\frac{d^2}{dx^2}\frac{1}{2}\psi + \frac{1}{2}m\omega^2 x^2 \psi$$

At this point, you should know what the above equation means. Just kidding! Don't worry, I have no idea what it means, but sometimes I leave these equations scribbled on pieces of paper on my desk so people think I'm really smart. The truth is that my career in mathematics unfortunately ended in high school because none of my instructors were able to impress upon me how amazing math really is. But now I know that every single thing in the universe, including the thoughts in our mind, can be broken down to mathematical equations such as the one above which translated means, "please stop talking about quantum physics!" Have no fear though, because after you understand all this, the rest of your day should be a piece of cake. Quantum physics is quite possibly the most complicated thing ever, even more so than the philosophy of the mind-body problem, so pat yourself on the back for even bothering to try and understand it. Another consolation is that you only need to understand the very basic concepts of quantum physics to appreciate how profound their impact can be. My explanations should be comprehendible to a fifth-grader (from 1952), or a present-day high-school sophomore.

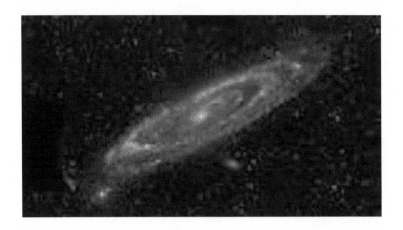

Since classical physics is the physics of big stuff, from the stuff that's big enough to see with our eyes down to the size of an atom, quantum physics is the physics of smaller stuff, that is, subatomic particles or particles that are smaller than atoms. It was previously believed that all physics should follow the same rules, but when you get down to subatomic particles, quantum physics throws the rules out the window. For example, one of the hallmarks of quantum physics is something called quantum entanglement. This occurs when two subatomic particles come in contact with each other and then are separated by any distance. When one of the particles is altered in some way after the two have separated, the other particle is effected in the exact same way, instantaneously, without any other influence whatsoever. This occurs regardless of the distance between the two particles, whether they're one inch or 186,000 miles apart. Quantum entanglement has been experimentally proven and generally accepted by mainstream science, yet it flies squarely in the face of classical physics because it defies Einstein's special theory of relativity. An instantaneous reaction will always be faster than the speed of light, but classical physics says nothing can travel faster than the speed of light because if it did than time would stop; but time doesn't stop for these quantum particles, so something is missing. Albert Einstein, not long after his discovery of the Special Theory of Relativity, stated that he was uncomfortable with quantum entanglement, calling it "spooky action at a distance" because it violated his own theories. The missing piece of the puzzle, the one that bridges the gap between the Special Theory of Relativity and quantum physics, is still missing. New research, however, is beginning to show that perhaps the answer to this puzzle lies in the mind. Trying to solve this mystery has given way to a new and controversial field called quantum consciousness, which proposes that consciousness cannot be explained in terms of classical physics alone, as it has been until now.

One of the problems with classical physics is that it implies that every single thing that happens in our lives is predetermined by a set of mathematical equations, and there are no other possible paths to take. In other words, it dictates that we can't change the course of our lives with our minds because we are destined to follow a classically predetermined path. However, quantum physics has opened the door to endless possibilities, giving us an opportunity to not only change our future, but potentially to change our past.

Collapse of The Wave Function

Nothing defines the infinite power of the mind more than the experience of having a eureka moment of sudden understanding. This is when you've been struggling with a problem for hours, days, or perhaps even years and suddenly, quite out of nowhere, the solution explodes into your mind. Have you ever wondered what exactly is happening in your mind to facilitate such an event, and whether it's possible to make it happen more often? New theories suggest that what's happening in your mind is something called the *collapse of the wave function*.

Quantum physics describes the world as we know it as a great ocean of information. This ocean holds all of the information in the universe, and before any information is transformed into a solid thought, experience, or piece of matter, it exists in the form of a wave, capable of being in an infinite number of locations, and capable of existing as an infinite number of possibilities, all at the same time. So every bit of information, every potential piece of anything exists everywhere simultaneously, and this is called *superposition*. Within this superposition, physicists define our potential reality by an equation they call "the wave function", depicted by the Greek letter psi, which is ironically the same symbol used to represent psychology, the unconscious, and parapsychology. If you look back at the quantum physics equation that I showed you before, you'll see it in there.

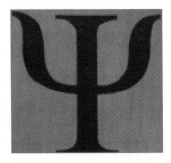

This *wave function* reflects all of the possible ways our potential information or piece of matter can evolve into an actual thought that we can comprehend consciously, or something that we can reach out and touch. Until the wave is observed in any way, it exists everywhere. But at the moment of any kind of observation, such as the act of measuring it or perhaps even just thinking about it, the wave function collapses into a single particle, a single thought, or a single experience, like an entire liquid ocean turning into a single molecule of water. Once the wave is observed and collapses into something we lay people would consider real and tangible, it sends shockwaves through the world as we know it, and changes everything. This has been scientifically proven to occur with subatomic particles, and proponents of quantum consciousness believe this process also takes place in the mind.

What's fascinating is that this *collapse of the wave function* cannot occur without something observing it, and the only thing capable of making an observation is a human consciousness. This is why classical physicists like Einstein resisted accepting these quantum theories, because to do so would be admitting that the human mind was far more powerful than they were comfortable with. What's even harder to believe is that quantum physics implies that nothing exists unless we are observing it. Einstein famously mocked this idea by asking if the moon was only there when he was looking at it, but the reality is that this might actually be the case.

*

Getting back to our eureka moment, quantum consciousness implies that all the knowledge that has ever entered our minds, consciously or unconsciously, and maybe even all of the knowledge in the universe, is available to us at any given moment, and that an infinite number of outcomes to the situation that you're pondering have the potential to become real. By simply asking a question in your mind, you're effectively creating the act of an observation of the wave function, causing it to collapse. This is the moment when the information crosses the barrier from quantum physics to classical physics and becomes conscious to you. If you're focused and tuned in enough during this process, it is possible that this universe of information can collapse into a single particle of knowledge, which takes the form of an answer to your question, and so now you have your "'Aha!" moment, and it feels like you've just been struck by lightning.

A good example of this process is when you ask a question on your computer and instantaneously all the information on the internet collapses to give you your answer. In fact, a large part of how a search engine and the internet works is based on quantum physics, and information technology companies must employ quantum physicists to make it all work so well.

*

It's difficult to comprehend just how powerful our minds are when we consider the potential of quantum consciousness combined with the powerhouse that lives inside our head. Consider that a human brain has one hundred billion brain cells, and each brain cell has up to forty thousand connections to other brain cells. If we do the math here, we will find that there are more connections in one human brain than there are stars in over forty thousand galaxies the size of our Milky Way. Daniel Amen gives us another example in his book, *Making A Good Brain Great*, when he describes how a piece of brain tissue the size of a grain of sand has one hundred thousand brain cells in it, with over a billion connections. So if you think you're incapable of doing something amazing with your life, you are grossly underestimating the power of your brain. Compared to the seemingly infinite knowledge and power of computers and the internet, each one of our brains has billions of more potential connections that are just waiting to be used or created, but most of it is just sitting there withering away from disuse. The few who have mastered their minds, by tapping into the universe of information surrounding them, and by practicing and disciplining their minds, over and over again, have learned that the more they do this, the more efficient their brains become, and the more "Aha!" moments they can have.

*

Quantum consciousness theories are far from being scientifically proven beyond a reasonable doubt, and there's no surprise how extremely controversial and hard to believe they are. But who would have believed that the internet would have been possible a century ago? Who would have believed that we would be able to land rovers on Mars? Accomplishing the successful landing of a rover on Mars was the equivalent, someone once said, of a person throwing a basketball from California and having it go through a hoop in New York, nothing but net.

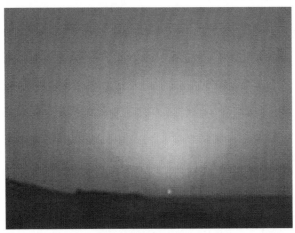

Sun setting on Mars

Quantum Physics is Everywhere

Quantum physics has found many applications in everyday life. It has allowed us to build transistors and lasers. Computers, MRI machines and the internet all work because humankind discovered the possibilities of the quantum world. Computer encryption relies on the equations of quantum physics which provide the highest security for the world's most sensitive information. Quantum teleportation, or the instantaneous transmission of information across space-time, has been experimentally verified with subatomic particles. It has also recently been discovered that photosynthesis is not governed by the laws of classical physics, as was previously thought, but by the mysterious rules of the quantum world; and without quantum physics, the sun wouldn't shine.

While I was doing my research, I was amazed at how long the proven theories of quantum physics have been around, how vast and amazing it makes the world we live in, and yet no one is really talking about this. Is it possible that we've been able to make quantum leaps with our minds all along, and that there's some sort of conspiracy to not let the cat out of the bag? Surely the world as we know it would cease to exist, the economy would collapse, and it would bring an end to capitalism if everyone knew about it, right? Hmm, I wonder. Surely, if this stuff was real, the government would know about it and be using it in many different ways, right?

ESP

Russell Targ is a physicist, author, and inventor who holds two NASA awards for inventions in lasers, and he cofounded the Stanford Research Institute's investigation into psychic abilities in the 1970s and 1980s. The U.S. government spent $20 million to fund this project which was controlled by the CIA. In his amazing book, *The Reality of ESP*, Mr. Targ discusses the relationship between quantum physics and ESP, and how the government used his research to train the military how to use something called remote viewing. Remote viewing was developed at Stanford Research Institute to enable people to describe and experience objects and events blocked from ordinary perception - often at great distances; it's a kind of ESP. Mr. Targ talks about how he conducted remote viewing experiments and training for the CIA for over twenty years. The CIA has only just recently declassified this information, so if you don't believe it you can look it up in the public domain, but I'm pretty sure they don't really want you poking around. This also left me thinking that if the CIA was doing this for 20 years, I can only imagine what else they've been doing.

Russell Targ also mentions another peculiar connection between ESP and the world of physics which occurred in the 1930s, around the same time that the theories of quantum physics were taking shape. Upton Sinclair (1878 -1968), one of the greatest American authors living at the time, wrote a book called *Mental Radio* in 1930, describing years of successful telepathic picture-drawing experiments that he carried out with his wife, Mary Craig. Albert Einstein was friends with Upton Sinclair and since they both lived in Princeton, New Jersey at the time of these experiments, Einstein had the opportunity to witness some of them. Einstein ended up writing the following preface to *Mental Radio*:

> The results of the telepathic experiments carefully and plainly set forth in this book stand surely beyond that which a nature investigator holds to be thinkable. On the other hand, it is out of the question in the case of so conscientious an observer and writer as Upton Sinclair that he is carrying on a conscious deception of the reading world; his good faith and dependability are not to be doubted. So if somehow the facts here set forth rest not upon telepathy, but upon some unconscious hypnotic influence from person to person, this also would be of high psychological interest. In no case should the psychologically interested circles pass over this book heedlessly. -- Albert Einstein May 23, 1930

The Sleeping Prophet

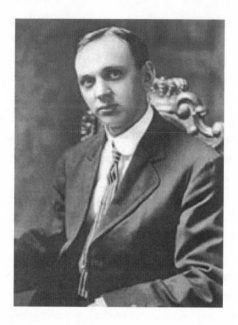

If anyone was ever able to tap into the infinite power of the mind, it was Edgar Cayce, a sweet and innocent man, living during the Great Depression, whose mind accidentally stumbled into another dimension. No matter where you stand on the issue of ESP, you'll take great joy in reading the biography of this amazing person, who has come to be known as one of the most famous psychics in history. He had the ability to answer questions about anything, from health and healing, to the outcome of wars, and the history of Atlantis. Edgar Cayce delivered his "life readings" to people while he was hypnotized, which gave him the nickname of "The Sleeping Prophet".

Edgar Cayce was born in 1877 and was the son of Kentucky tobacco farmers with only an eighth-grade education. As a child, the psychic abilities that he began displaying were things such as seeing auras around people, speaking to angels, and hearing voices of departed relatives. He also said that he was able to memorize entire books by leaving them next to his pillow while he slept. His parents dismissed this as an overactive imagination, which left Edgar confused as to what to make of it all.

Despite his eighth-grade education, Edgar ultimately developed the ability to diagnose and treat physical and mental conditions by hypnotically channeling an entity which he called "The Source". During his lifetime, he gave 14,145 fully documented readings for 5,744 people with over 170,000 pages of supporting documentation. Edgar not only gave readings on medical ailments, he answered questions on the future, the past, the stock market, and Jesus Christ. He became a national celebrity and gave readings to the most prominent people in the world at the time, such as Thomas Edison, Nikola Tesla, Irving Berlin, Marilyn Monroe, and Nelson Rockefeller to name a few. There's even circumstantial evidence that he did a reading for President Woodrow Wilson while he was still in office. Edgar Cayce has also been credited with helping develop the FM radio.

Edgar Cayce insisted on giving readings to people free of charge. He asked for voluntary donations to support himself and his family so that he could give readings full-time. To help raise money, he invented a card game called "Pit", based on commodities trading at the Chicago Board of Trade. The game was produced by Parker Brothers in 1903. Allegedly, the only thing Cayce ever got out of it was a check for six dollars from Parker Brothers and a dozen decks of the cards; the game is still sold today by Parker Brothers.

Edgar was noted to have said that everyone has access to this power, and that the unconscious mind has access to information that the conscious mind does not. Edgar also said that the most important thing that people can do to facilitate this ability is to be a more spiritual and loving person, which would enable them to "bring light to a waiting world".

A Little Bit More About Quantum Physics

The most conceivable explanation for the powers of Edgar Cayce's mind is surely embedded in the quantum world. Many people find stories like Cayce's hard to believe, but consider a few more quantum situations that have been scientifically proven at a subatomic level, and perhaps are happening in our macroscopic world as well.

-The Observer effect refers to the fact that it is not possible to observe a system without changing the system in some way. In experiments with electrons, the act of measuring the path that an electron takes will fundamentally change the outcome of the experiment. So theoretically, everything you look at, touch, or think about is changed by you in some way, hopefully for the better.

-The quantum zeno effect, proven in an experiment by Cornell physicists, is the ability to suspend the time evolution of an unstable particle by continuously observing it. This prevents the particle from decaying as it would in the absence of that observation; and as we already know, the only thing capable of making an observation is a human consciousness. It's fascinating to think that, in some deep recesses of our universe, it is possible to stop the evolution of time with our minds. If this effect reaches into the mechanisms of our daily lives, think of the implications it can have. Paying attention to something can keep it from dying.   •

-Bell's theorem, supported by a substantial amount of experimental evidence, states that an invisible stream of energy will always connect any two objects that have been connected in any way in the past. Imagine if this applies to everyone you've ever come in contact with.

As I was finishing writing this book, China launched the first quantum satellite, making hack proof communication possible for the first time ever. This was such an amazing feat that it has left the United States decades behind China in the realm of quantum technology. This event can also be compared in significance to the Soviet Union being the first country to launch a man into space, which was plastered all over the front page of every newspaper, but no one's really talking about China's satellite now because most people don't have any idea what quantum physics is all about.

*

A fascinating difference between the way most people think things are, and the way the quantum world is, is discussed by Stephen Hawking and Leonard Mlodinow in their book, *The Grand Design*. Consider a particle that is moving from point A to point B. Most people would think the that particle will take a definitive path to get from point A to point B, but the quantum reality is that the particle can take every possible path, all at the same time. If the particle looks back at point A to see the path that it took, it could see a different path other than the one it actually took. The implications of this are astounding because this means that the past may not be set in stone like we thought it was. Hawking and Mlodinow state, "Quantum physics tells us that no matter how thorough our observation of the present, the (unobserved) past, like the future, is indefinite and exists only as a spectrum of possibilities. The universe, according to quantum physics, has no single past, or history". If the effects of quantum physics can somehow reach into our macro world, this could mean that our own personal history is not fixed, and that the things we do in the present can not only affect our future, but can also change our past. One exception to this rule might apply to killing yourself though. I'm not sure if even quantum physics can save you then because once you've killed yourself, you won't be around in the future to have any effect on the past, which is one more reason not to kill yourself. But assuming you haven't thrown yourself off a bridge yet, if you make a mistake, you could conceivably improve the outcome of it even after it has already happened, based on your response afterward.

*

Much of the latest information about quantum physics has been discovered by experiments conducted inside of a particle accelerator in Europe called the Large Hadron Collider or LHC. LHC is a massive 27-

kilometer-long ring structure of superconducting magnets, tunnels, coils, cables and computers. The greatest experimental physicists in the world use this collider to smash particles into each other at close to the speed of light, to try and learn more about our universe. Some of the information they get will ultimately determine whether or not we live in a parallel universe, or in a multiverse. In other words, it has already been accepted by many of the leading scientists of the world that there is more than one universe, and possibly millions more... imagine that.

Faith of A Mustard Seed

Since I've gone so far as to link quantum physics to parallel universes, ESP, mind-reading, and hypnotic channeling, why stop there? A talk about the infinite potential of the mind would not be complete without a discussion about psychokinesis. Okay, I know this sounds crazy, but even Jesus told his disciples that if they had faith the size of a mustard seed they could uproot a tree. And besides, it's fun to talk about moving things with your mind, and how do you know it's not possible?

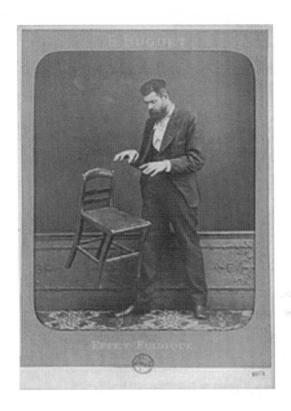

Psychokinesis refers to the mind changing matter without any other form of energy being responsible. In their research paper entitled, "Biological Utilization of Quantum Nonlocality", Nobel Prize laureate Brian Josephson and coauthor Fotini Pallikara-Viras proposed that explanations for both psychokinesis and telepathy might be found in quantum physics. Dean Radin, the controversial researcher and chief scientist at the Institute of Noetic Sciences (IONS), also believes that perhaps the quantum world gives us evidence to support the existence of psychokinesis and other such phenomena. He discusses these concepts in *The Conscious Universe* and *Entangled Minds*.

Many people throughout history have claimed to have the ability to move things with their minds, and just about everyone thinks they're crazy because this ability has never been proven to actually exist in our macro world. But if quantum physics gives us the ability to move a subatomic particle by observing it, then why is it crazy to think that we can move mountains as well?

Coral Castle

Moving matter with the mind is not a new concept; it has possibly been around for thousands of years. There are many famous ancient monolithic building sites all over the world, and in many cases, scientists have been greatly challenged to explain how people were able to build them. Maybe the ancient people knew how to move mountains with their minds and the secret has long been lost; most would disagree, but attempts to reproduce the construction of these structures using only the limited tools that were available at the time have been questionable at best. These structures were built thousands of years ago with stones weighing in some cases hundreds of tons, cut, stacked, and placed so close together that light could not even pass through. The pyramids of Giza, Stonehenge, and the site at Puma Punku in Bolivia are amazing examples. I was also fascinated to learn that there was a much more recent and mysterious monolithic building site right here in the United States.

The American monolith story is about a man named Edward Leedskalnin, a Latvian immigrant who was born in 1887 to a family of stonemasons. As the story goes, Edward's sixteen-year-old fiancée broke up with him in Latvia, just one day before their wedding. Heartbroken, he decided to go to the United States where he built a monument to his long-lost love. He was a solitary man who never married and spent the rest of his life building what has come to be known as Coral Castle. It's made of monolithic stone structures that Edward, five feet tall and only weighing one hundred pounds, allegedly built and moved by himself with his own hands and without any cranes or lifts. It still stands there today on South Dixie Highway near the city of Homestead, Florida and belongs to the U.S. National Register of Historic Places.

Edward spent almost three decades of his life building Coral Castle. The grounds consist of over 1,000 tons of stones that were formed into walls, doors, carvings, furniture and a castle tower. Most objects were made from single pieces of stone weighing fifteen tons on average. The stones fit together so well that no light passes through the joints, and without the use of mortar, they have stayed perfectly in place for decades.

Edward was very private, and supposedly refused to allow anyone to view him while he worked. The only tool that he mentioned using was a "perpetual motion holder", and he said this worked by a process called reverse magnetism. The source of this power was allegedly created by a black box suspended from a tripod that was placed over the stones that he wanted to move.

Edward charged visitors ten cents a person to tour the castle grounds. When asked why he had built the castle, he would vaguely answer that it was for his "Sweet Sixteen". Billy Idol also wrote the song *Sweet Sixteen* after visiting Coral Castle.

Many people dispute the claim that Edward built Coral Castle mysteriously by himself, and they say that he did it the old-fashioned way: with blood, sweat, tools and tears. However he did it though, I'll bet that quantum physics was somehow involved. Coral Castle remains a popular tourist attraction today and as the story goes, when questioned about how he moved the large stones, Edward would reply that he "understood the laws of weight and leverage well" and that he had "discovered the secrets of the pyramids".

*

Most people don't believe in all this paranormal stuff, but it is peculiar how a select few of some of the most amazing people who have ever lived, do believe in it. Robert Cialdini, Ph.D., one of the most influential social psychologists of this century talks about what he did before he was a famous social psychologist in his best-selling book, *Pre-Suasion*. He was a palm reader, and one of his explanations for his success at this credits "paranormal mechanisms that can be mastered fully by only a select few."

Magnetoreception

Maybe you can't move mountains with your mind, but perhaps you have a better sense of direction than other people. Another mind-boggling effect of quantum physics is something called magnetoreception. We've all been at a fork in the road in life and had to choose which way to go. Sometimes there's no fork at all, and we're just in the middle of a forest with no path in sight. Some of us are better than others at sensing which way is the right way to go; we are somehow drawn in the right direction. Is it possible that there is an invisible force helping guide us on our journey? Recent biological discoveries may offer some insight.

Magnetoreception is the sense by which many insects and animals are able to detect a magnetic field to help them figure out where they are or where they're going. Homing pigeons have long been considered to have this ability, but now we know that bees, butterflies, dolphins, sharks, and sea turtles, among many other things, also have this ability. By looking at satellite pictures, one researcher discovered that even grazing cows align themselves toward the magnetic north pole. The mechanism for how this works is linked to quantum entanglement and the quantum Zeno effect, which makes the functioning of atomic magnetometers possible. Magnetite has been located in the beaks of pigeons, and magnetite nanoparticles have been found in the heads of rainbow trout. There's a growing body of evidence suggesting that humans may also have magnetoreceptive abilities, because magnetic particles have also been found in human nasal bones. More evidence in support of magnetoreception in humans is the discovery of a magnetosensitive protein called cryptochrome-2 in the retina of the eye. Cryptochrome could potentially create a type of visual compass within us, allowing us to see the earth's magnetic field, in a similar way that we can see heat waves emanating off the road on a hot summer day.

It's not hard to imagine that if all of these insects and animals possess this ability, that we do too. This gives more meaning to the idea of being drawn to something we love, and repelled by things we dislike. By keeping ourselves tuned into our own internal compass, we will stay on course and avoid falling into the miserable abyss that so many lost souls find themselves in.

The Butterfly Effect

I feel so much better than I did when I started this journey, but I haven't forgotten that the potential to slip back into chaos will always exist for me, and despite how far I've come, and with all that I have to be thankful for, I can still easily remember what it was like to not look forward to another cold tomorrow. Every now and then, but with tragic regularity, a movie star or a rock star jumps off a bridge, hangs themselves, drowns in a bathtub, or overdoses on pain medication. When the person who dies is someone who has touched me in some way, I always feel like a small part of me dies with them. Many of these deaths are suicides that shock the world, while at the same time thousands of other people take their lives with little or no fanfare. Maybe it's not too late to save some of them.

Many of the 43,000 people that will kill themselves this year probably think that their life is unfolding predictably and uncontrollably before them; and that, ultimately, nothing they say or do really matters in the grand scheme of things. If we could only get these people to see that even a very small positive change in their thinking can result in arbitrarily large deviations from their predicted behavior. Then they would know that the tiniest positive thought could make them reconsider their choice to jump, make them step back from the edge, and decide to give life another chance.

How could something so small make such a big difference? One explanation lies in what has come to be known as the butterfly effect, one of the subjects of chaos theory. The idea is that something even as small as the flap of a wing from a butterfly could cause a chain reaction leading to a hurricane years later, or as Stephan Hawking has said in his famous book, *The Universe In a Nutshell,* "A butterfly could flap its wings in Tokyo and cause it to rain in New York."

*

Someday, everyone will appreciate how powerful our minds can be, and that our possibilities really are endless. It's unfortunate that the latest technological advances have done little, if anything, to improve the quality of our mental health, but maybe it's not too late. There's still a chance for quantum consciousness research to help us find better ways to feel better. In the meantime, I will continue to try and tap into the infinite potential of my own mind by practicing using all the tools that have kept me headed in the right direction.

As I watch my daughter grow up, I think of myself when I was her age and sometimes yearn to go back in time to help the lost little girl that I used to be. I guess in a sense, that is what I have done. By writing this book and doing all this work on myself, maybe I was able to go back in time to throw that little girl a lifeline and pull her through the tough times.

As I have become a better person now, my daughter will also be a better person; and maybe she will change the world, because I told her she could. I will also teach her everything that I wish I had known when I was younger. She will know that life, especially the present moment, is a precious gift. She will know that if her source of light comes from within herself, then no one else can put it out, and she can share this light with the world, and use it to explore the universe in all its wonder. She will know that her mind is a powerful instrument, and that it can be as destructive as it is creative, and that she must continuously channel its energy in a positive direction. She will know that she can do anything she dreams of if she puts her heart and soul into it, and she will know that everything she thinks, says, or does sets off a chain reaction of events that will forever change the course of her life.

*

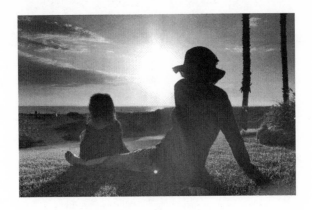

For so long now, we have allowed the chaos in the world and the chaos in our minds to poison our hearts and souls, but maybe it's time to change. Maybe it's time to believe in something a little more meaningful, something a little more magical. Maybe then we can get that feeling back again, the one we used to have all the time as a child; whether we were just sitting on the porch, or playing in the rain, the feeling was always with us. We can find our way back to that special place again, and when we do we'll realize that it was here all the time, just waiting for us to come back. This is what I was missing all along...this is where I went wrong. I thought that the best part of my life had passed me by, but I can see it now, and it's sitting right in front of me.

I have often said that *easy* is boring, but every now and then, it's nice when life is easy. Once we master our minds and close the gap between what we have and what we want, then can we take a walk down easy street. Some people will want to know how we got there, so we must show them the way. Once they find their path, then they can show others, and the process can keep repeating itself until it spreads across the globe. I can't think of a greater gift to give a child, or a friend, than the knowledge that if a butterfly can change the world, so can they.

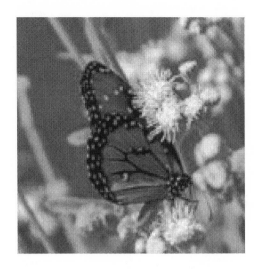

THE END

I hope this book, however imperfect it may be, has made you think about life in a different and perhaps more interesting way; after all, it's the thought that counts.

NOTES

On the cover see "Image of the day gallery, Star Cluster NGC 2074" 8/11/08, nasa.gov. Credit: NASA, ESA, and Hubble Heritage Team (STScl/AURA). Web. 10 January 2015.
Chapter 1
For the quote "only that day dawns to which we are awake" see brainyquote.com. 4 September 2013.
For the picture of Golden Gate Bridge, see Golden Gate Bridge = File: Golden Gate Bridge, HAER CA-31-47.jpg. commons.m.wikimedia.org. Web. 17 February 2015.
On the Golden Gate Bridge shoe display discussion and the fact that the number of suicides has risen 31% see Martin, Timothy W. "Middle-Aged Suicides Surge." *The Wall Street Journal* 3 May 2013: A1. Print.
On the most popular spots to commit suicide see Oliveri, Denise, "Bridge Of Death-Suicides At The Golden Gate Bridge." *JuniorDr.* n.d. Web. 25 August 2014 and "Nanjing Yangtze Suicide Bridge." *Weird Asia News.* 25 January 2007. Web. 12 August 2014.
On the history of suicides at the Golden Gate Bridge see Starr, Kevin. *Golden Gate: the life and times of America's greatest bridge.* New York: Bloomberry Press, 2010. 165-169. Print. Bateson, John, "The Suicide Magnet that is the Golden Gate Bridge." *LA Times,* 29 September 2013. Web. 25 August, 2014. "1000th Succumbs To Morbid Allure Of Golden Gate Leap." *Desert News.* Associated Press, 11 July 1995. Web. 18 December 2013. Adams, Jane Meredith. "Golden Gate Bridge Suicides Reach 1,000 And Counting". *The Baltimore Sun.* 12 July 1995. Web. 2 August 2014. Pogash, Carol, "Suicides Mounting, Golden Gate Looks to Add a Safety Net." New York Times, 8 May 2014. Web. 7 July 2014. Libman, Joan. "Golden Gate Bridge: Triumph, Tragedy: Suicide Rate Shadows the Span's 50th Anniversary Celebration." Los Angeles Times, 22 May 1987. Web. 18 June 2014.
On Sarah Rutledge Birnbaum see "Woman Survives Golden Gate Bridge Fall," apnewsarchive.com. Associated Press, 2 January 1988. Web. 18 August 2014. Beedle, Carolyn Clark. "Bridging History, Tragedy and Celebration." Beyond Doorways Travel. n.d. Web. 26 August 2014.
For the image of "The Street Girl's End" see commons.wikimedia.org.
For the statistics on veteran suicides see Carney, Jordain. "Why Are So Many Older Veterans Committing Suicide?" nationaljournal.com , 4/13/2014. Web. 19 February 2015.
For the student survey on suicide conducted by the CDC see "Suicide Prevention-Youth Suicides" Centers for Disease Control and Prevention, cdc.gov January 9, 2014. Web. 2/26/2015.
On the statistics about suicides and the number of suicides rising 31% in the last decade see CDC.gov/suicide, NIH.gov/suicide.
For quote "no one can learn to be at home in his own heaven, until he learns to be at home in his own hell" see Presnall, Lewis F. *Search For Serenity.* Salt Lake City, Utah: U.A.F., 1959. 1. Print.
The mental health statistics of adults and children was found on the National Alliance of Mental Illness "Mental Illness Facts and Numbers" sheet at nami.org, 27 August 2014.
On the 12 deadliest shootings see Klein, Ezra. "Twelve facts about guns and mass shootings in the United States". *The Washington Post.* Wonkblog. 14 December 2013. Web. 18 January 2014.
Regarding studies showing antidepressants aren't any better than placebo see Weil, Andrew M.D. *Spontaneous Healing.* New York: Little, Brown and Comapny, 2011. 53. Print. Harvard Mental Health Letter, "Treating social anxiety disorder." Volume 26 Number 9, March 2010. Harvard Health Publications (2010): 3. print. Insel, Thomas. "Director's Blog: Antidepressants: A Complicated Picture." 12/6/11. nimh.nih.gov. National Institute of Mental Health. Web. 19 February 2015.
For the statistics on antidepressant use in the United States see *"Antidepressant Use in Persons Aged 12 and older: United States, 2005-2008".* Centers for Disease Control and Prevention, October 2011. Web. 3 March 2013.
For the facts about valium see Cooper, Arnie, *"An Anxious History of Valium."* The Wall Street Journal, 15 November 2013. Web. 4 January 2014. Herper, Matthew, "America's Most Popular Mind Medicines." forbes.com. 17 September 2005. Web. 5 November 2014.

On the Nietzsche quote, "Man is the only animal who needs to be encouraged to live" see Tanzi, Rudolph E. and Chopra, Deepak. *Superbrain: Unleashing the Explosive Power of Your Mind to Manage Health, Happiness, and Spiritual Well-Being.* New York: Harmony Books, 2012. 153. Print.

For Pericles' quote "With us it is no disgrace to be poor; the true disgrace to doing nothing to avoid poverty" see Gross, Ronald. *Socrates' Way: Seven Keys to Using Your Mind to the Utmost.* New York: Jeremy P. Tarcher/Putnam, 2002. 5. Print.

For the discussion on how the normal state of the mind is chaos see Csikszentmihalyi, Mihaly. *Flow: The Psychology Of Optimal Experience.* New York: Harper Perennial Modern Classics, 2008. 119. Print.

On discussion of negative thoughts see Harris, Russ. *The Happiness Trap.* Boston: Trumpeter Books, 2007. 43. Print. Markway, Barbara Ph.D. *"Stop Fighting Your Negative Thoughts."* Psychology Today. 7 May 2013. Web. 4 October 2013.

The image of Rich Koz as the Son of Svengoolie is reprinted with permission and courtesy of Rich Koz/MeTV.

On the mental health statistics of US population see "U.S. Adult Mental Illness Surveillance Report," cdc.gov. Centers for Disease Control and Prevention, 7 September 2011. Web. 5 September 2014.

On a discussion of 'flow' and the 'gap' between what we want and what we have and controlling one's consciousness see Csikszentmihaly, Mihaly. *Flow: The Psychology of Optimal Experience.* New York: Harper Perennial Modern Classics, 2008. 243,20. Print.

Chapter 2

The image of The Thinker is from Wikipedia contributors. "The Thinker." Wikipedia, The Free Encyclopedia. Wikipedia, The Free Encyclopedia, 9 May. 2014. Web. 4 Sep. 2014.

Bruce Lee quote see "as you think, so shall you become." brainyquote.com n.d. Web. 2 September 2014.

For the image of Albert Einstein see commons.wikimedia.org/wiki/File:Einstein_patentoffice.jpg

On the discussion of Albert Einstein's brain see Isaacson, Walter. *Einstein: His Life and Universe.* New York: Simon & Schuster, 2007. 545-548. Print. "The Exceptional Brain of Albert Einstein." lifescience.bioquant.com. Bioquant Life Science, n.d. Web. 18 February 2014.

For the definitions of the mind, think, and consciousness see Merriam-Webster's Collegiate (R) Dictionary, 10th Edition, 1999. "mind", 740; "think", 245, "consciousness", 1226.

For the Oracle of Delphi see "The Oracle at Delphi." pbs.org. PBS, n.d. Web. 24 May 2013. Spiller, Henry A., John R. Hale, and Jelle Z. de Boer. "The Delphic Oracle: A Multidisciplinary Defense of the Gaseous Vent Theory." *Clinical Toxicology* 40.2, 2000. 189–196. Web. 24 May 2013. Roach, John. "Delphic Oracle's Lips May Have Been Loosened by Gas Vapors". news.nationalgeographic.com *National Geographic, 14 August 2001.* Web. 5 May 2013. "The Oracle of Delphi," coastal.edu, n.d. Web. 6 November 2014.

For the images of the remaining columns of the Temple of Apollo see Wikipedia contributors. "Temple of Apollo." Wikipedia, The Free Encyclopedia. On the Oracle of Delphi and the King of Lydia see Gross, Ronald. *Socrates' Way.* New York: Jeremy P. Tarcher/Putnam, 2002. 82-84. Print.

For the image of "Priestess of Delphi" see Wikipedia contributors. "Pythia." Wikipedia, The Free Encyclopedia. Wikipedia, The Free Encyclopedia, 25 Jul. 2014. Web. 4 Sep. 2014.

For the image of Socrates see "Socrates", wpclipart.com, web, 19 January 2015.

For the image of "The Death of Socrates" see Wikipedia contributors. "The Death of Socrates." Wikipedia, The Free Encyclopedia. Wikipedia, The Free Encyclopedia, 9 Jan. 2015. Web. 19 Jan. 2015.

For the story of Socrates' friend asking the Oracle if there's any man wiser than Socrates see Gross, Ronald. *Socrates' Way.* New York: Jeremy P. Tarcher/Putnam, 2002. 82-83. Print.

For the following quote "Happy is he who knows that he knows nothing, or next to nothing, and holds his opinions like a bouquet of flowers in his hand, that sheds its fragrance everywhere, and which he is willing to exchange at any moment for one fairer and more sweet, instead of strapping them on like an armor of steel and thrusting with his lance those who do not accept his notions" see Willard, Frances, *A Wheel Within A Wheel.* New York: Revell Company, 1895. 43-44. Print.

On the discussion and definition of the Socratic Method see Jarratt, Susan C. *Rereading the Sophists: Classical Rhetoric Refigured.* Carbondale and Edwardsville: Southern Illinois University Press, 1998. 22, 83,84. Print. "The Socratic Method." law.uchicago.edu. The University of Chicago Law School, n.d. Web. 4 September 2014.

Maxwell, Max, "Introduction To The Socratic Method and it's Effect on Critical Thinking." socraticmethod.net. n.d. Web. 7 November 2014.

For the discussion about asking the right questions see Gross, Ronald. *Socrates' Way.* New York: Jeremy P. Tarcher/Putnam, 2002. 58,73. Print.

Chapter 3

On the discussion of the id, ego, and superego see Meyerhoff, Michael K. "Delayed Gratification". *Pediatrics for Parents* Volume 23 Issue 1 (2007): 8-9. Print. "Pieces Of The Mind, In Conflict", *Secrets of Genius* (2004): 29, *U.S. News & World Report* (2004).

Kaplan, Harold I. M.D. and Benjamin J. Sadock, M.D. *Kaplan And Sadock's Synopsis of Psychiatry* Eighth Edition. Baltimore, Maryland: Williams and Wilkins, 1998. 217-222. Print.

For the quote by Freud, "the ego is like a man on horseback..." see McLeod, Saul. "Id, Ego, and Superego." simplepsychology.org. SimplePsychology, 2008. Web. 4 September 2014.

For a discussion on the distinction between narcissism and narcissistic personality disorder see Twenge, Jean M. Ph.D. and W. Keith Campbell, Ph.D. *Living In the Age of Entitlement: The Narcissism Epidemic.* New York: Free Press, 2009. 22. Print.

For statistics of narcissistic personality disorder see "Any Personality Disorder." nimh.nih.gov. National Institute of Mental Health, 2007. Web. 5 September 2014. "1 in 5 Young Americans Has Personality Disorder." nbcnews.com. Associated Press, 1 December 2008. Web. 5 September 2014. "Narcissistic Personality Disorder." mentalhealth.com. Internet Mental Health, n.d. 24 July 2014.

For description of the narcissistic individual see Moore, Thomas. *Care Of The Soul: A Guide For Cultivating Depth And Sacredness In Everyday Life.* New York: HarperPerennial, 1992. 72-75. Print. "Narcissistic Personality Disorder." mayoclinic.org. Mayo Clinic, n.d. Web. 2 August 2014.

For the image of Narcissus by Caravaggio see Wikipedia contributors. "Narcissism." Wikipedia, The Free Encyclopedia. Wikipedia, The Free Encyclopedia, 3 Sep. 2014. Web. 5 Sep. 2014.

On the myth of Narcissus see Seautan, Gnotti. "Legend." echo.me.uk. n.p. 30 April 2008. Web. 11 March 2013. "The myth of Narcissus." greekmyths-greekmythology.com. n.d. Web. 2 May 2013.

On the discussion of the clinical characteristics of narcissistic individuals and clinical advice on treatment see Kaplan, Harold I. M.D. and Benjamin J. Sadock, M.D. *Kaplan And Sadock's Synopsis of Psychiatry* Eighth Edition. Baltimore, Maryland: Williams and Wilkins, 1998. 213-217. Print. Twenge, Jean M. Ph.D. and W. Keith Campbell, Ph.D. *Living In the Age of Entitlement: The Narcissism Epidemic.* New York: Free Press, 2009. 20, 29. Print. Benjamin, Lorna Smith Ph.d. *Interpersonal Diagnosis and Treatment of Personality Disorders, 2nd Edition.* New York: Guilford Press, 1996. 142-146. Print. Hahn, Rhonda K., Lawrence J. Albers, M.D., and Christopher Reist, M.D., *Psychiatry*, 1997 Edition. Laguna Hills, CA: Current Clinical Strategies Publishing, 1997. 64-66. Print.

For the study on the prevalence of NPD see Stinson, Frederick S. Ph.D, Deborah A. Dawson, Ph.D., [...] and Bridget F. Grant, Ph.D."Prevalence, correlates, disability, and comorbidity of DSM-IV Narcissistic Personality Disorder". ncbi.nlm.nih.gov. The Journal of Clinical Psychiatry, July 2008. 69(7): 1033-1045. Web. 7 September 2014.

Chapter 4

On Joe Simpson's ordeal and Touching the Void see *Touching The Void.* Dir. Kevin Macdonald. John Smithson, 2003. Netflix. 6 September 2012.

On overcoming adversity see Csikszentmihaly, Mihaly. *Flow: The Psychology of Optimal Experience.* New York: Harper Perennial Modern Classics, 2008. 90-92.

For the quote by Friedrich Nietzsche "That which does not kill us makes us stronger" see brainyquote.com. n.d. Web. 5 September 2014.

On the quote about Martin Seligman's positive psychology see Weil, Andrew M.D. *Spontaneous Healing.* New York: Little, Brown and Company, 2011. 130.Print.

Chapter 5

For statistics on video game usage see "How Much Do You Know About Video Games?" esrb.org. Entertainment Software Rating Board, n.d. Web. 9 September 2014. Esterl, Mike. Amount of time children play video games, *Wall Street Journal,* June 2013. A3. Print. "Youth Risk Behavior Surveillance - United States 2013." cdc.gov. Web. 13 June 2014.

On the discussion of flow see Nakamura, Jeanne and Mihaly Csikszentmihalyi. "The Concept of Flow." n.d. mywebstewdwards.edu. Web. 16 April 2015. Csikszentmihaly, Mihaly. *Flow: The Psychology of Optimal Experience.* New York: Harper Perennial Modern Classics, 2008.58, 71-73, 162. Print. Cherry, Kendra. "What Is Flow?", psychology.about.com, n.d. Web. 20 April 2015.

For the statistics on drug addiction see Hafner, Josh, *Surgeon general: 1 in 7 to suffer addiction, USA Today,* November 18-20, 2016.

For the image of Vincent van Gogh see Wikipedia contributors. "Vincent van Gogh." Wikipedia, The Free Encyclopedia. Wikipedia, The Free Encyclopedia. For the image of Jeanne Louise Calment see Wikipedia contributors. "Jeanne Calment." Wikipedia, The Free Encyclopedia. Wikipedia, The Free Encyclopedia, 16 Jan. 2015. Web. 19 Jan. 2015. On Jeanne Louise Calment's story see "World's oldest person dies at 122." cnn.com. CNN, 4 August 1997. Web. 10 February 2014. "World's Oldest Person Dead", *McCook Daily Gazette,* August 4, 1997, Volume 74 Number 29 Section One.

Chapter 6

For the statistics on how often people cry see "Women cry more often than men, and for longer, study finds." telegraph.co.uk. The Telegraph, 15 October 2009. Web. 8 September 2014.

For why we cry see "On the Origin of Crying and Tears." froes.dds.nl. Human Ethology Newsletter, Vol 5 Issue 10, June 1989, p 5-6. Web. 9 September 2014.

On the discussion of Chauvet Cave see Herzog, Werner. *"Cave of Forgotten Dreams."* Dir. Werner Herzog, 2010. Netflix. 3 March 2012. For the images of Chauvet Cave see Wikipedia contributors. "Chauvet Cave." Wikipedia, The Free Encyclopedia. Wikipedia, The Free Encyclopedia, 29 Jul. 2014. Web. 8 Sep. 2014.

For the statistics on how much people watch TV see "A Look Across Screens, The Cross-Platform Report." iab.net, Q12013NeilsenCrossPlatformReport.pdf. Web. 2 April 2012. Regarding the Bureau of Labor Statistics and almost 91 million people over the age of 16 not working see "Labor force statistics from the current population survey", data.bls.gov. Web. 13 October 2014.

On the number of drowning deaths in Australia see Barlass,Tim and staff writers. "Number of drowning deaths amongst toddlers increasing." essentialbaby.com.au. Essential Baby, 8 December 2013. Web. 16 June 2014.

For the story about the shooting death of Justin Valdez see Daily Mail Reporter, "San Francisco rail passengers were so absorbed in their phones and tablets, they didn't notice a man waving a gun before he randomly shot dead a commuter." 8 October 2013, dailymail.co.uk. Web. 22 February 2015.

For the image of the Gettysburg Address see Wikipedia contributors. "Gettysburg Address." Wikipedia, The Free Encyclopedia.

For the discussion of handwriting and the quote "Millennials can't read cursive" see Gasparo, Annie. "Whole Foods Plans New Store Concept." *The Wall Street Journal,* B1,B7. Print. 7 May 2015.

Chapter 7

For the image of cavemen see "Diorama, caveman - National Museum of Mongolian History.jpg." commons.wikimedia.org. 31 December 2012. Web. 14 August 2013.

For the discussion on the shrinking of human brains see McAuliffe, Kathleen. "If Modern Humans Are So Smart, Why Are Our Brains Shrinking?"; discovermagazine.com. Discover, 20 January 2011. Web. 19 June 2013. Holloway, April. "Scientists are alarmed by shrinking of the human brain." 14 March 2014. ancient-origins.net. Web. 3 Feb 2015.

On the statistics of Alzheimer's Disease see "Alzheimer's Facts and Figures." alz.org. Alzheimer's Association, 2014. Web. 8 September 2014.

For the statistics on anxiety in America and less developed countries see McBain, Sophie. "Anxiety Nation." *New Statesman* 4/11/2014, Vol. 143 Issue 5205, p. 24-27.

On the discussion of intelligence and IQ see "Analytical Intelligence: Definition, Lesson & Quiz", education-portal.com, n.d. Web. 4 December 2014. Gladwell, Malcolm. *Outliers: The Story of Success.* New York: Little, Brown and Company, 2008. 77-80. Print.

For the classification of IQ see "The Measurement And Appraisal of Adult Intelligence: David Wechsler: Free Download & Streaming: Internet Archive." archive.org. n.d. Web. 12 April 2013.

For the Robert J. Baum study on practical intelligence see Society for Industrial and Organizational Psychology (SIOP). "High level of practical intelligence a factor in entrepreneurial success." sciencedaily.com. ScienceDaily, 30 October 2010. Web. 4 January 2013.

For Robert J. Baum's quote on practical intelligence see Baum, J. Robert. "The Practical Intelligence of High Potential Entrepreneurs." www-old.rhsmith.umb.edu. Smith School of Business - University of Maryland, n.d. 5 September 2014.

On the discussion of practical intelligence and Robert Sternbergs definition of it and on the general discussion of IQ see Gladwell, Malcolm. *Outliers: The Story of Success.* New York: Little, Brown and Company, 2008. 101, 78-80. Print. Sternberg, R.J. *Beyond IQ: A Triarchic Theory of Intelligence.* Cambridge: Cambridge University Press, 1985.

On the discussion of life expectancy in the US see Tavernise, Sabrina. "Life Spans Shrink for least educated whites in US." nytimes.com. New York Times, 20 September 2012. Web. 18 February 2013.

For the image of Plato see Wikipedia contributors. "Plato." Wikipedia, The Free Encyclopedia. Wikipedia, The Free Encyclopedia, 9 Oct. 2014. Web. 9 Oct. 2014.

On the allegory of "The Cave" see On the discussion of The Allegory of the Cave see "The Allegory of the Cave." faculty.washington.edu. n.d. Web. 9 October 2014. Pearcy, Mark. "The Allegory of the Cave by Plato: Summary, Analysis and Explanation. education-portal.com. n.d. Web. 7 January 2015. Barlow, Dudley. "The Teacher's Lounge." *Education Digest.* Mar 2008, Vol 73 Issue 7, p. 67-71. Gross, Ronald. *Socrates' Way: Seven Keys to Using Your Mind to the Utmost.* New York: Jeremy P. Tarcher/Putnam, 2002. 116-119. Print.

For the statistic on 29% of the world population being obese see McKay, Betsy. "About 29% of World Is Overweight." *The Wall Street Journal:* A6, 30 May 2014. Print.

For the discussion and quotes regarding prescription pain killer overdoses see "Policy Impact: Prescription Painkiller Overdoses." cdc.gov. Centers for Disease Control and Prevention, 2 July 2013. Web. 9 October 2014.

For the discussion on experts spending 10,000 hours perfecting their skill see Gladwell, Malcolm. *Outliers: The Story of Success.* New York: Little, Brown and Company, 2008. 38,39,42. Print. Ericsson, K. A. (2006). Protocol analysis and expert thought: Concurrent verbalizations of thinking during experts' performance on representative task. In K. A. Ericsson, N. Charness, P. Feltovich, and R. R. Hoffman, R. R. (Eds.). Cambridge handbook of expertise and expert performance (pp. 223-242). Cambridge, UK: Cambridge University Press.

For the discussion on being alone see Csikszentmihaly, Mihaly. *Flow: The Psychology of Optimal Experience.* New York: Harper Perennial Modern Classics, 2008. 119,168-169. Print.

For exploring your fear see Csikszentmihaly, Mihaly. *Flow: The Psychology of Optimal Experience.* New York: Harper Perennial Modern Classics, 2008. 43. Print.

For taking action in your life see McGraw, Phillip C. Ph.D. *Life Strategies: Doing What Works, Doing What Matters.* New York: Hyperion 1999. 127.Print.

Chapter 8

For the quote "Misery is optional" see Presnall, Lewis F. *Search For Serenity.* Salt Lake City, Utah: U.A.F., 1959.v. Print.

For the quote by Carl Jung see Wallace, Sebastian. "What you resist will persist." wallacearticles.blogspot.com. Philosophy of Psychology. 10 October 2010. Web. 8 September 2014.

For the statistics on anxiety disorders and the clinical definition of generalized anxiety disorder and symptoms see "Anxiety Disorders." nimh.nih.gov. National Institute of Mental Health, n.d. Web. 6 July 2013. "Generalized Anxiety Disorder." mayoclinic.org. Mayo Clinic, 8 September 2011. Web. 17 September 2014.

For the discussion on 'errors in logic' see Kaplan, Harold I. M.D. and Benjamin J. Sadock, M.D. *Kaplan And Sadock's Synopsis of Psychiatry* Eighth Edition. Baltimore, Maryland: Williams and Wilkins, 1998. 623-625, 921. Print.

For the image of the Titanic see Wikipedia contributors. "RMS Titanic." Wikipedia, The Free Encyclopedia. Wikipedia, The Free Encyclopedia, 11 Jan 2015. Web. 22 January 2015.

On the discussion of the payoffs that people get from their anxiety see Firestone, Robert Ph.d. "How to Stop Playing the Victim Game." psychologytoday.com. 30 April 2013. Web. 4 August 2014. Boyes, Dr. Alice. "Why You Keep Doing Things You Hate: Understanding Unwanted Behavior Patterns." Psychology for Everyday Life. n.d. Web. 16 October 2014. McGraw, Phillip C. Ph.D. *Life Strategies: Doing What Works, Doing What Matters.* New York: Hyperion 1999. 88.Print.

On the discussion about social anxiety see "Social Anxiety." webmd.com. 8 December 2014. Jacobs, Andrew M. Psy.D. and Anthony M. Martin. Phd. "Social Anxiety and Social Phobia." socialanxietysupport.com. Social Anxiety Support, n.d. Web. 4 November 2013.

On the discussion of the four choices of how to respond in a difficult social encounter see Beck, Aaron T., Gary Emery, Ph.D., and Ruth Greenberg, Ph.D. *Anxiety Disorders And Phobias*, 15th Edition. Cambridge, MA: Basic Books, 2005. 284-285. Print.

Quote by Dr. Seuss, "those who mind don't matter, and those who matter don't mind," see Falconer, Ian. *Dream Big (Olivia).* Kansas City, MO: Andrews McMeel Publishing, 2006. 14. Print.

On the general discussion of treating anxiety, cognitive behavioral therapy, and acknowledging painful emotions see "What to do about social anxiety disorder." Harvard Women's Health Watch, Volume 16 Number 16 December 2008, pg 3. Kaplan,

Harold I. M.D. and Benjamin J. Sadock, M.D. *Kaplan And Sadock's Synopsis of Psychiatry* Eighth Edition. Baltimore, Maryland: Williams and Wilkins, 1998.581.Print. Beck, Aaron T., Gary Emery, Ph.D., and Ruth Greenberg, Ph.D. *Anxiety Disorders And Phobias*, 15th Edition. Cambridge, MA: Basic Books, 2005. 167, 177, 238. Print. Borysenko, Joan Ph.D. with Larry Rothstein. *Minding the Body, Mending the Mind.* Reading, MA: Addison-Wesley Publishing Company, 1988. 37. Print.

For the quote "The past is history..." see *Kung Fu Panda*, youtube.com, 14 December 2014.

For practicing being "the eye of the storm" see Carlson, Richard Ph.D. *Don't Sweat The Small Stuff...and it's all small stuff.* New York: Hyperion, 1997. 155. Print.

For the image of Hurricane Katrina see File:Katrina-noaaGOES12.jpg at en.wikipedia.org. Web. 22 September 2014.

For the discussion on breathing see Weil, Andrew M.D. *Spontaneous Healing.* New York: Little, Brown and Company, 2011.146.Print.

On answering the 'what ifs' see Beck, Aaron T., Gary Emery, Ph.D., and Ruth Greenberg, Ph.D. *Anxiety Disorders And Phobias*, 15th Edition. Cambridge, MA: Basic Books, 2005. 201, 208. Print.

For the painting "The Gulf Stream" see Wikipedia contributors. "The Gulf Stream (painting)." Wikipedia, The Free Encyclopedia. Wikipedia, The Free Encyclopedia, 30 May. 2014. Web. 14 Sep. 2014.

For the discussion of Debbie Downer see "Debbie Downer Thanksgiving Dinner/ Saturday Night Live - Yahoo Screen." screen.yahoo.com. 14 September 2014.

On negative thinking see Jeffrey Ph.D. and Susan Magee. *Why Can't You Read My Mind.* New York: Marlowe & Company, 2004. 54. Print.

For the quote "For every minute you're angry you give up sixty seconds of peace of mind" see brainyquote.com. 14 September 2014.

For the discussion of how some people have a lower threshold for getting angry than others see Svitil, Kathy A. *Calming The Anger Storm.* Indianapolis, IN: Alpha Books, 2005. 6. Print.

On what happens when people get angry see Bernstein, Jeffrey Ph.D. and Susan Magee. *Why Can't You Read My Mind.* New York: Marlowe & Company, 2004. 156. Print.

Regarding the discussion of the word "anger" being the first thing seen onscreen see "The Incredible Hulk", imbd.com. 8 December 2014.

On the discussion of flooding see Goleman, Daniel. *Emotional Intelligence.* New York: Bantam Books, 1995. 61,139. Print.

For unrealistic expectations triggering our rage see McGraw, Phillip C. Ph.D. *Life Strategies: Doing What Works, Doing What Matters.* New York: Hyperion 1999. 168.Print.

On the discussion of domestic violence in the US see domesticviolencestatistics.org. Domestic Violence Statistics, n.d. Web. 3 September 2014.

For the quote "the explosive force of gasoline..." see Presnall, Lewis F. *Search For Serenity.* Salt Lake City, Utah: U.A.F., 1959. 114-115. Print.

For the quote "holding onto anger is like grasping a hot coal..." see brainyquote.com. 14 September 2014. Borysenko, Joan Ph.D. with Larry Rothstein. *Minding the Body, Mending the Mind.* Reading, MA: Addison-Wesley Publishing Company, 1988. 170. Print.

For the discussion of considering the consequences of our actions before we act them out see Branden, Nathaniel. *Honoring The Self: Self-Esteem And Personal Transformation.* New York: Bantam Books, 1985. 83-84. Print.

On the idea of acting how someone amazing you know would act and how being thankful makes it more difficult to be angry see Svitil, Kathy A. *Calming The Anger Storm.* Indianapolis, IN: Alpha Books, 2005. 37, 207. Print.

For the image of a brain cell see Wikipedia contributors. "Neuron." Wikipedia, The Free Encyclopedia. Wikipedia, The Free Encyclopedia, 14 Sep. 2014. Web. 15 Sep. 2014.

On the discussion of how studies have shown changes in the brain after psychotherapy see Karlsson, Hasse MA, MD, Phd. "How Psychotherapy Changes the Brain", Psychiatric Times, psychiatrictimes.com, 8/11/11. Web. 20 August 2015.

On the discussion of bad brain pathways verses good brain pathways see Doidge, Norman M.D. *The Brain That Changes Itself.* New York: Penguin Books, 2007. 209-211. Print.

On the discussion of what we can do to alleviate our fears see Beck, Aaron T., Gary Emery, Ph.D., and Ruth Greenberg, Ph.D. *Anxiety Disorders And Phobias*, 15th Edition. Cambridge, MA: Basic Books, 2005.278-279. Print.

Chapter 9

For the discussion of fear see Solomon, Andrew; *Mental Illness Is Not A Horror Show, The New York Times,* October 26, 2016; nytimes.com. *Bloodcurdling movies and measure of coagulation: Fear Factor crossover trial;* BMJ 2015;351:h367.

For the discussion of the amygdala see "Amygdala." sciencedaily.com, n.d. 10 Decmeber 2014. Baily, Regina. "Amygdala." biology.about.com, n.d. 10 Decmeber 2014. O'Brien, Ginny. "Understanding Ourselves: Gender Differences in the Brain." columbiaconsult.com, The Columbia Consultancy, Volume #52, Fall 2007. Yandell, Kate. "Scaring Those Who Have No Fear." the-scientist.com, 5 February 2013. Kaplan, Harold I. M.D. and Benjamin J. Sadock, M.D. *Kaplan And Sadock's Synopsis of Psychiatry* Eighth Edition. Baltimore, Maryland: Williams and Wilkins, 1998. 93-94. Print. Lloyd, Robin, "Emotional Wiring Different in Men and Women." livescience.com. LiveScience, 19 April 2006. Web. 22 September 2014. Markowitsch HJ. "Differential contribution of right and left amygdala to affective information processing." ncbi.nlm.nih.gov. National Institute of Health, 1998. Web. 18 August 2014. Goleman, Daniel. *Emotional Intelligence*. New York: Bantam Books, 1995. 15-18. Print. Nadler, Dr. Relly. "What Was I Thinking? Handling the Hijack." psychologytoday.com. and truenorthleadership.com. July 2009. Web. 4 October 2013.

For the images of Navy Seals see sealswcc.com. For image of Navy Seals underwater see Wikipedia contributors. "United States Navy SEALs." Wikipedia, The Free Encyclopedia. Wikipedia, The Free Encyclopedia, 19 Jan. 2015. Web. 20 Jan. 2015.

On the discussion of the Navy Seals mental training process see "Navy Seals Mental Training Video." youtube.com. video segment uploaded on 15 February 2012 from "The Brain" documentary featured on the History Channel. Web. 6 March 2014.*The Brain*. Dir. Richard Vagg, November 10, 2008, The History Channel. Akil II, Bakari Ph.D. "How the Navy Seals Increased Passing Rates." psychologytoday.com. Psychology Today, 9 November 2013. Web. 9 December 2013.

For the discussion of reappraisal see Aamodt, Sandra Ph.D and Sam Wang. *Welcome To Your Brain*. New York: Bloomsbury, 2008. 104-106. Print. Troy, Allison S., Frank Hl Wilhelm, [...], and Iris B. Mauss, "Seeing the Silver Lining: Cognitive Reappraisal Ability Moderates the Relationship Between Stress and Depressive Symptoms. National Institutes of Health, ncbi.nlm.nih.gov. 10 Dec 2010. Web. 27 April 2015. Goleman, Daniel. *Destructive Emotions*. New York: Bantam Books, 2004. 145. Print.

Chapter 10

For the image of "The Premature Burial" see Wikipedia contributors. "Premature burial." Wikipedia, The Free Encyclopedia. Wikipedia, The Free Encyclopedia, 6 Aug. 2014.

Chapter 11

For the discussion of psychological visibility see Branden, Nathaniel. *The Six Pillars of Self-Esteem*. New York: Bantam Books, 1995. 180, Print. Branden, Nathaniel. *The Psychology of Romantic Love*. New York: Bantam Books, 1981. 82-83, 154-155. Print.

On the discussion of how The Little Prince does not get psychological visibility from the 'grown-ups' see Saint Exupery, Antoine de. *The Little Prince*. New York: Harvest/HBJ, 1943, 1971. 4. Print.

For the quote by Mark Twain "Forgiveness is the fragrance a violet sheds on the heel that has crushed it" see brainyquote.com. Web. 22 September 2014.

For the quote and discussion on being the first person to do the understanding and being a better listener see Carlson, Richard Ph.D. *Don't Sweat The Small Stuff...and it's all small stuff*. New York: Hyperion, 1997. 213,73, 76. Print.

For the quote "a man convinced against his will is of the same opinion still" see Carnegie, Dale. *How To Win Friends and Influence People*. New York: Pocket Books, 1936. 111. Print.

On the discussion on talking too much and how the goal of communication is not to win a battle, and to avoid bringing up old baggage see Bernstein, Jeffrey Ph.D. and Susan Magee. *Why Can't You Read My Mind*. New York: Marlowe & Company, 2004. 131, 155. Print.

On shifting the balance by being the first person to understand see Borysenko, Joan Ph.D. with Larry Rothstein. *Minding the Body, Mending the Mind*. Reading, MA: Addison-Wesley Publishing Company, 1988. 141. Print.

For the quote "even the lowest whisper can be heard - over armies, when it's telling the truth" see "The Interpreter (2005) Quotes." imdb.com. IMDb, n.d. Web. 22 September 2014.

On the discussion about John Gottman and his research on how couples interact and the behaviors and facial expressions most predictive of divorce see gottman.com. Gladwell, Malcolm. *Blink: The Power of Thinking Without Thinking*. New York: Little, Brown and Company, 2005.20-24, 32-33. Print.

For the discussion of Paul Ekman and facial expressions see paulekman.com. *"The Psychology Book: Big Ideas Simply Explained."* Contributors: Catherine Collin, Nigel Benson, and Joannah Ginsburg. New York: DK Publishing, 2012. 196-197. Print. Gladwell, Malcolm. *Blink: The Power of Thinking Without Thinking*. New York: Little, Brown and Company, 2005. 204. Print. Goleman, Daniel. *Destructive Emotions*. New York:

Bantam Books, 2004. 120-122. Print. On Paul Ekman's research revealing a link between facial expressions and our nervous system see Goleman, Daniel. *Destructive Emotions*. New York: Bantam Books, 2004. 130. Print.

Chapter 12

On how hormones in your diet increase your risk of getting cancer see Plant, Jane A. *Your Life In Your Hands: Understand, Prevent, and Overcome Breast Cancer and Ovarian Cancer*. New York: Thomas Dunne Books, 2000. Print.

For a discussion of Dr. Andrew Weil's website, vitamins, dietary supplements see drweil.com.

For the discussion of radiation, uranium, superfund sites, and radon see epa.gov. Regarding the statistics and symptoms of autism see "Autism Spectrum Disorder (ASD) Data & Statistics." cdc.gov. Centers of Disease Control and Prevention, 24 March 2014. Web. 4 June 2014.

Regarding the statistics and symptoms of attention deficit/hyperactivity disorder see "Attention Deficit/Hyperactivity Disorder (ADHD) Data & Statistics." cdc.gov. Centers For Disease Control and Prevention, 13 November 2013. Web. 4 June 2014.

For the discussion on the first nuclear reactor built and where it was buried see Kamps, Kevin. "Red Gate Woods: History's First Radioactive Dust Bin." beyondnuclear.org. Beyond Nuclear, 1 December 2012. Web. 23 September 2014. Enshwiller, John R. and Jeremy Singer-Vine. "A Nuclear Cleanup Leaves Questions Lingering at Scores of Old Sites." *The Wall Street Journal*, 30 October 2013. Print.

For the image of the monument that sits on top of the burial site of the first nuclear reactor see the U.S. Department of Energy or pruned.blogspot.com. Web. 22 January 2015.

On the statistics of superfund sites in Alabama and New Jersey see "superfund sites where you live." epa.gov. Web. 23 September 2014

For the statistics of ADHD in New Jersey and Kentucky see Holland, Kimberly and Elsbeth Riley, "ADHD by the Numbers: Facts, Statistics, and You" September 4, 2014. healthline.com. 13 December 2014.

Chapter 13

On the discussion of humor being the number two trait for mates see Lippa RA. "The preferred traits of mates in a cross-sectional study..." ncbi.nlm.nih.gov. April 2007. Web. 10 July 2014.

For the quote from research conducted by the National Institute of Health, "humor involves the ability to detect incongruous ideas violating social rules and norms...and requires a complex array of cognitive skills for which intact frontal lobe functioning is critical." see "humor and the brain", nih.gov. n.d. Web. 23 September 2014.

For the discussion on how humor works in the brain see Aamodt, Sandra Ph.D and Sam Wang, *Welcome To Your Brain*. New York: Bloomsbury, 2008. 105. Print. Brain, Marshall. "How Laughter Works." science.howstuffworks.com. n.d. Web. 24 September 2014.

Chapter 14

For the quote by Arthur Schopenhauer see brainyquote.com.

On the discussion of bisociation see Koestler, Arthur. *The Act of Creation*. New York: Penguin Books, 1964. 13, 29, 38. Print. Dubitzzky et al. "Towards Creative Information Exploration- Based on Koestler's Concept of Bisociation", link.springer.com. Bisociative Knowledge Discovery, Lecture Notes in Computer Science Volume 7250, 2012, pp. 11-32. On how Koestler believes "people are most creative when rational thought is suspended" and most people's creativity is "frequently suppressed by the automatic routines..." see Keostler, Arthur. *The Act of Creation*. New York: Penguin Books, 1964. Back Cover. Print.

For the discussion of how creativity was viewed originally see Simonton, Dean Keith Ph.d. "The Psychology of Creativity: A Historical Perspective." psychology.ucdavis.edu. n.d. web. 14 December 2014.

On the IBM survey of CEO's see "Creativity Selected as Most Crucial Factor for Future Success." www-03.ibm.com. 18 May 2010. Web. 25 September 2014.

On the discussion of creativity and the brain see Drexel University. *"Brain Activity Differs For Creative and NonCreative Thinkers."* sciencedaily.com. ScienceDaily, 29 October 2007. Web. 25 September 2014. Lehrer, Jonah. *Imagine: How Creativity Works*. New York: Houghton Mifflin Harcourt Publishing Company, 2012. 32-33. Print.

For the discussion of convergent vs. divergent thinking see "Strategies of Divergent Thinking." faculty.washington.edu. n.d. web. 14 December 2014. Lehrer, Jonah. *Imagine: How Creativity Works*. New York: Houghton Mifflin Harcourt Publishing Company, 2012. 64-65. Print

On Einstein's solution to the Theory of Relativity being revealed to him in a dream see Bhagirathananda. *My Yanja: Recollections, Notes and Essays*. Quills Ink Publishing, 2014.

On the statement of Charles Darwin's father accusing him of being lazy and too dreamy see Michalko, Michael. "Famous Failures." creativitypost.com. The Creativity Post. 11 May 2012. Web. 25 September 2014.

On Graham Wallas's five stages of the creative process see Wallas, Graham. *Art of Thought*. Kent, England: Solis Press, 1926, 2014. 38-42. Print. Popova, Maria. "The Art of Thought: Graham Wallas on the Four Stages of Creativity, 1926." brainpickings.org. n.d. 14 December 2014.

For Robert Goddard having his ideas rejected by his peers see Michalko, Michael. "Famous Failures." 11 May 2012. Web. 25 September 2014.

For the discussion on the link between mood disorders and creativity see Andreasen, Nancy C., MD, PhD. "The relationship between creativity and mood disorders." ncbi.nlm.nih.gov. n.d. Web. 15 December 2014. Roberts, Michelle. "Creativity 'closely entwined with mental illness' ". 17 October 2012. bbc.com. BBC News Health, web, 15 December 2014.

On how alpha waves increase creativity see Bergland, Christopher. "Alpha Brain Waves Boost Creativity and Reduce Depression." psychologytoday.com/blog. April 17, 2015. Web. 11 May 2015. Lehrer, Jonah. *Imagine: How Creativity Works*. New York: Houghton Mifflin Harcourt Publishing Company, 2012. 30-31. Print.

For colors effect on attention to detail and creativity see University of British Columbia. "Effect of Colors: Blue Boosts Creativity, While Red Enhances Attention To Detail." sciencedaily.com. ScienceDaily, 6 February 2009. Web. 31 March 2014.

On how exercise increases creativity see Burns, Will. "Multiple Creativity Studies Suggest: Creating Our Reality Requires Detaching From It." forbes.com. 10 July 2013. Web. 20 April 2015. Bergland, Christopher. "The Neuroscience of Imagination: Aerobic Exercise Stimulates Creative Thinking Post", psychologytoday.com/blog. Feb 8, 2012. Web. 11 May 2015.

Regarding the 1950's rat experiments on the pleasure centers of the brain see Kurzweil, Ray. "*How To Create A Mind: The Secret Of Human Thought Revealed.*" New York: The Penguin Group, 2012. 105. Print.

For the discussion on uncertainty see Chopra, Deepak. *The Seven Spiritual Laws of Success*. San Rafael, CA: Amber-Allen Publishing, 1993. 86-87. Print.

Chapter 15

For the quote "Narcissus falls in love with his image, but he doesn't know it is he that is loved" see Moore, Thomas. *Care Of The Soul: A Guide For Cultivating Depth And Sacredness In Everyday Life*. New York: HarperPerennial, 1992. 73. Print.

For the image of the painting *Narcissus* by Caravaggio see Wikipedia contributors. "Narcissus (mythology)." Wikipedia, The Free Encyclopedia. Wikipedia, The Free Encyclopedia, 25 September 2014.

For the definition of self-esteem and the discussion of perseverance see Branden, Nathaniel. *The Six Pillars of Self-Esteem*. New York: Bantam Books, 1995. 4. Print. Branden, Nathaniel. *Honoring The Self: Self-Esteem and Personal Transformation*. New York: Bantam Books, 1985. 46. Print.

For a further discussion of self-esteem as well as the attributes of people with high and low self-esteem see Reasoner, Robert. "The True Meaning Of Self-Esteem", The National Association for Self-Esteem, self-esteem-nase.org, 4/27/15. Web. "Self-Esteem", University of Texas Counseling and Mental Health Center, utexas.edu/, Web. 27 April 2015. Branden, Nathaniel. *Honoring The Self: Self-Esteem and Personal Transformation*. New York: Bantam Books, 1985. 8-9. Print.

For the image of the painting of George Washington crossing the Delaware see Wikipedia contributors. "Washington Crossing the Delaware." Wikipedia, The Free Encyclopedia. Wikipedia, The Free Encyclopedia, 28 Aug. 2014. Web. 25 Sep. 2014.

On Jung's view of self and a discussion of projection see Jung, Carl G. (editor), *Man And His Symbols*. New York: Dell Publishing, 1964. 163, 169, 174, 267 (mandala).

For the discussion of projection and low self-esteem see Kaplan, Harold I. M.D. and Benjamin J. Sadock, M.D. *Kaplan And Sadock's Synopsis of Psychiatry* Eighth Edition. Baltimore, Maryland: Williams and Wilkins, 1998. 220, 519. Print.

Regarding projection in relationships see Eigen, Rebeca E. "*Is It Love Or Is It Projection? The Anima/Animus Phenomenon*". shadowdance.com. n.d. Web. 17 December 2014.

For the discussion of codependence see Sun, Feifei. "Are You in a Codependent Relationship?". webmd.com. WebMD, n.d. Web. 25 September 2014. Hahn, Rhonda K., Lawrence J. Albers, M.D., and Christopher Reist, M.D., *Psychiatry*, 1997 Edition. Laguna Hills, CA: Current Clinical Strategies Publishing, 1997.67-68. Print.

For the discussion of bad boundaries see Collins, Bryn C. M.A., L.P. *Emotional Unavailability*. Chicago: Contemporary Books, 1997. 68. Print. Schafer, Jenny, "5 Signs You Might Have Bad Boundaries" 5/28/13, herscoop.com. Web. 26 December 2014.

On the psychology of codependence see Forward, Susan. *Obsessive Love: When It Hurts Too Much To Let Go.* New York: Bantam Books, 1991. 172-174, 187. Print. Branden, Nathaniel. *Honoring The Self: Self-Esteem and Personal Transformation.* New York: Bantam Books, 1985. 37-38. Print. "Savior Complex Anyone?" peopleskillsdecoded.com. n.d Web. 25 September 2014. Claire, Barbara. "Looking At Unconscious Compulsions in Our Relationships." heartlinks2spiritualwellness.com. n.d. Web. 25 September 2014.

On reparenting see McGraw, Phillip C. Ph.D. *Life Strategies: Doing What Works, Doing What Matters.* New York: Hyperion 1999. 208.Print.

Chapter 16

For the discussion of Martin Seligman and his research on learned helplessness see Kaplan, Harold I. M.D. and Benjamin J. Sadock, M.D. *Kaplan And Sadock's Synopsis of Psychiatry* Eighth Edition. Baltimore, Maryland: Williams and Wilkins, 1998. 163. Print. Cherry, Kendra. "What Is Learned Helplessness." psychology.about.com. About Education, n.d. 27 September 2014. Borysenko, Joan Ph.D. with Larry Rothstein. *Minding the Body, Mending the Mind.* Reading, MA: Addison-Wesley Publishing Company, 1988. 22-23. Print.

Regarding the studies showing learned helplessness in humans and animals see Hiroto, Donald S. and Martin E. Seligman. "Generality of learned helplessness in man." Journal of Personality and Social Psychology, February 1975. psycnet.apa.org. American Psychological Association. Web. 27 September 2014.

On the quote by Dr. Laura Markham on how children will "create new brain pathways to talk themselves through difficult situations in the future" see Markham, Laura. "8 Steps to Help Your Child Develop Self-Control." ahaparenting.com. Aha!parenting.com, n.d. Web. 4 February 2015.

For the discussion of "The Marshmallow Test" see Mischel, Walter; Ebbesen, Ebbe B. and Antonette Raskoff Zeiss. "Cognitive and attentional mechanisms in delay of gratification." psycnet.apa.org. American Psychological Association, February 1972.

On the discussion of "The Marshmallow Test" and children building brain pathways associated with self-discipline see Markham, Laura. "8 Steps to Help Your Child Develop Self-Control." ahaparenting.com. Aha!parenting.com, n.d. Web. 27 September 2014.

On the discussion of how 71% of young adults are rejected by the military see Jordan, Miriam. "Uncle Sam Wants You-Unless You're 71% of Youths." *The Wall Street* Journal: A1, A5. 28 June 2014. Print.

Chapter 17

For the image of the astronaut see Wikipedia contributors. "Astronaut." Wikipedia, The Free Encyclopedia, 12 Sep. 2014.

Regarding how many employees really like their jobs, see McGregor, Jenna; *Only 13 percent of people worldwide actually like going to work; The Washington Post;* October 10, 2013; washingtonpost.com.

For the "Earthrise" image see "Earthrise at Christmas". nasa.gov. NASA, n.d. Web. 27 September 2014.

For the quote "As a day well spent procures a happy sleep, so a life well employed procures a happy death" by Leonardo Da Vinci see "What You Find Meaningful." manifestyourpotential.com. n.d. Web. 29 September 2014.

For the quote by Dolly Parton, "I hope to fall over dead onstage right in the middle of a song", see "Your Looking Swell Dolly" by Amy Maclin, The Oprah Magazine, June 2016, 112.

For the term "life deferral" plan and how the "math doesn't work" see Ferriss, Timothy. *The 4-Hour Workweek.* New York: Crown Publishers, 2007. 279, 31. Print.

On how nothing shrinks the brain more than doing the same thing over and over see Doidge, Norman M.D. *The Brain That Changes Itself.* New York: Penguin Books, 2007. 87, 256. Print.

For the discussion on how "You have to name it to claim it" see McGraw, Phillip C. Ph.D. *Life Strategies: Doing What Works, Doing What Matters.* New York: Hyperion 1999. 210.Print.

Chapter 18

For the discussion of brain plasticity see Doidge, Norman M.D. *The Brain That Changes Itself.* New York: Penguin Books, 2007. 20-23,213. Print. Cherry, Kendra. "What Is Brain Plasticity?", psychology.about.com, n.d. Web. 20 April 2015.

For the discussion of how increased stress and depression can kill brain cells see Gregoire, Carolyn. "How Stress Changes The Brain." huffingtonpost.com, 11/18/2014. Web. 6 April 2015.

On the things to do to exercise your brain see "Exercise Your Brain". Your Brain Matters - The Power of Prevention. yourbrainmatters.org.au. n.d. Web. 27 February 2015. Doidge,

Norman M.D. *The Brain That Changes Itself*. New York: Penguin Books, 2007. 251, 254. Print

Chapter 19

On the discussion of how visualizing yourself doing some activity strengthens the muscles used in that activity see Quinn, Elizabeth. "Visualization and Muscle Strength." sportsmedicine.about.com. May 17, 2013. Web. 8 April 2015.

On the process of visualization and improving mental imagery see Weil, Andrew M.D. *Spontaneous Healing*. New York: Little, Brown and Company, 2011. 145. Print.

On learning from our mistakes without making them see Gilbert, Daniel. *Stumbling on Happiness*. New York: Alfred A. Knopf, 2006. 138. Print.

For the discussion of negative mental imagery see Morina, Nexhmedin, Catherine Deeprose, [...], and Emily A. Holmes, "Prospective mental imagery in patients with major depressive disorder or anxiety disorders." Journal of Anxiety Disorders, 2011 December, National Institutes of Health, ncbi.nlm.nih.gov. Web. 28 April 2015. Beck, Aaron T., Gary Emery, Ph.D., and Ruth Greenberg, Ph.D. *Anxiety Disorders And Phobias*, 15th Edition. Cambridge, MA: Basic Books, 2005. 213. Print.

Chapter 20

On the ancients and dreams see Crisp, Tony. "Egyptian (ancient) Dream Beliefs." dreamhawk.com. n.d. 7 January 2015. Web.

On why we forget our dreams see Hartman, Ernest. "Why Do Memories of Vivid Dreams Disappear Soon After Waking Up?" scientificamerican.com. 14 April 2011. Web. 7 January 2015.

Regarding Kekule dreaming about the structure of benzene see Penrose, Roger. *The Emperor's New Mind*. New York: Oxford University Press, 1989. 546. Print.

Regarding Einstein dreaming about E=mc2 and the special theory of relativity see "Albert Einstein." dreaminterpretation.com. n.d. Web. 3 May 2014.

For the discussion of how sleeping and dreaming improve the processing of information and learning see Wansley, Erin J. Ph.D and Robert Stickgold, Ph.D. "Memory, Sleep and Dreaming: Experiencing Consolidation." National Institutes of Health. ncbi.nlm.nih.gov. 3/1/2011. Web. 10 April 2015.

Chapter 21

For the discussion on dualism and the mind-body problem see Penrose, Roger. *The Emperor's New Mind*. New York: Oxford University Press, 1989. 27, 205, 523. Print.

For the discussion of dualism see Robinson, Howard, "Dualism", The Stanford Encyclopedia of Philosophy (Winter 2012 Edition), Edward N. Zalta (ed.), URL = <http://plato.stanford.edu/archives/win2012/entries/dualism/>. Calef, Scott. "Dualism and Mind". iep.utm.edu. n.d. Web. 7 January 2015.

For the image of Descartes see Wikipedia contributors. "René Descartes." Wikipedia, The Free Encyclopedia. Wikipedia, The Free Encyclopedia, 9 Oct. 2014. Web. 9 Oct. 2014.

On the discussion of monism see Schaffer, Jonathan, "Monism", The Stanford Encyclopedia of Philosophy (Winter 2014 Edition), Edward N. Zalta (ed.), forthcoming URL = <http://plato.stanford.edu/archives/win2014/entries/monism/>.

For the discussion of the Phineas Gage story see Twomey, Steve. "Phineas Gage: Neuroscience's Most Famous Patient." smithsonianmag.com. Smithsonian Magazine, January 2010. Web. 9 October 2014. Aamodt, Sandra and Sam Wang. *Welcome To Your Brain*. New York: Bloomsbury USA, 2008. 170. Print.

For the image of Phineas Gage see File: Phineas Gage GageMillerPhoto2010-02-17 Unretouched Color Cropped.jpg. commons.m.wikimedia.org. Web. 22 January 2015.

On the discussion of how Cartesian dualism caused mainstream science to believe that the brain was fixed and unchangeable see Doidge, Norman M.D. *The Brain That Changes Itself*. New York: Penguin Books, 2007. 213-214. Print.

For the discussion of the mind-body problem and free will see "Henry Stapp." informationphilosopher.com. Information Philosopher, 5 May 2013.

For the image of Isaac Newton see Wikipedia contributors. "Isaac Newton." Wikipedia, The Free Encyclopedia. Wikipedia, The Free Encyclopedia, 9 Oct. 2014. Web. 10 Oct. 2014.

Regarding quantum entanglement see Vergano, Dan. "'Spooky' Quantum Entanglement Reveals Invisible Objects." news.nationalgeographic.com. National Geographic, 27 August 2014. Web. 9 October 2014. Brooks, Michael. "How Weird Do You Want It?" *New Scientist*. 9/13/2014, Vol 223 Issue 2986, p. 34-37.

For the image of the Andromeda galaxy see "Andromeda." jpl.nasa.gov . Courtesy NASA/JPL- Caltech. Web. 4 October 2014.

For the discussion on quantum consciousness see quantumconsciousness.org. Also see "Henry Stapp." informationphilosopher.com. Information Philosopher, 5 May 2013.

On the collapse of the wavefunction see "Wave Function Collapse." princeton.edu. n.d. Web. 6 October 2014. Anderson, Mark. "Is Quantum Mechanics Controlling Your Thoughts?" discovermagazine.com. 13 January 2009. *What the Bleep Do We Know?*, Directors: William Arntz, Betsy Chasse, Mark Vicente, April 2004. "Henry Stapp." informationphilosopher.com. Information Philosopher, 5 May 2013. Penrose, Roger. *The Emperor's New Mind.* New York: Oxford University Press, 1989. 524-525, 560. Print. Tolson, Jay. "Is There Room for the Soul?" *U.S. News & World Report*, 10/23/2006, Vol 141 Issue 15, p. 56-63. Tegmark, Max. "Many lives in my worlds" *Nature*, 7/5/2007, Vol 448 Issue 7149, p. 23-24.

For the discussion of having an 'Aha! moment' see Penrose, Roger. *The Emperor's New Mind.* New York: Oxford University Press, 1989. 541-544. Print.

For the statistics on the number of brain cells and connections see Amen, Daniel G. *Making A Good Brain Great.* New York: Harmony Books, 2005. 20. Print.

On the discussion on where quantum physics is found such as in photosynthesis see Anderson, Mark. "Is Quantum Mechanics Controlling Your Thoughts?" discovermagazine.com. 13 January 2009.

For the discussion of Russell Targ and his work at the Stanford Research Institute in relation to remote viewing and the CIA see Targ, Russell. *The Reality of ESP.* Wheaton, IL: Quest Books, 2012. Back cover, 42-45, 201-202. Print.

On the discussion of Albert Einstein writing the preface to Upton Sinclair's book *Mental Radio* as well as the preface itself see Targ, Russell. *The Reality of ESP.* Wheaton, IL: Quest Books, 2012. 232. Print. "Full Text of *Mental Radio.*" archive.org n.d. Web. 11 October 2014. Sinclair, Upton. *Mental Radio.* Springfield, Illinois: Charles C. Thomas Publisher, 1930. Preface. Web. 11 October 2014.

For the discussion of Edgar Cayce see Kirkpatrick, Sidney D. *Edgar Cayce: An American Prophet.* New York: Riverhead Books, 2000. 9-11,27-30,88-91,102- 103, back cover. Print.

For the discussion on quantum zeno effect and quantum entanglement see Zimmerman Jones, Andrew. "Quantum Zeno Effect," and "What Is Bell's Theorum." physics.about.com. about education, n.d. 11 October 2014. Physics and Consciousness, *Quantum Interconnectedness*, starstuffs.com. "Henry Stapp." the informationphilosopher.com. The Information Philosopher, n.d. Web. 2 August 2014.

Regarding the launching of China's quantum satellite, see Chin, Josh – "China Makes A Quantum Leap Forward", The Wall Street Journal, 16, August, 2016.

For the observer effect see Weizmann Institute Of Science. "Quantum Theory Demonstrated: Observation Affects Reality." ScienceDaily. ScienceDaily, 27 February 1998. <www.sciencedaily.com/releases/1998/02/980227055013.htm>.

For the discussion of how a particle takes every path possible simultaneously and how history is not fixed see Hawking, Stephen and Leonard Mlodinow. *The Grand Design.* New York: Bantam Books, 2010. 75, 82. Print.

Regarding the Large Hadron Collider see "About CERN", home.web.cern.ch.

For the image of psychokinesis see Wikipedia contributors. "Psychokinesis." Wikipedia, The Free Encyclopedia. Wikipedia, The Free Encyclopedia, 9 Oct. 2014. Web. 16 May 2014.

For the statement by Jesus to his disciples that if they had the faith of a mustard see they could uproot a tree see *Good News Bible.* New York: American Bible Society, 1976. Luke 17:6. Print.

Regarding the research conducted by Nobel Prize laureate Brian Josephson see Josephson, Brian D. and Fontini-Pallikara-Viras. "Biological Utilisation of Quantum Nonlocality." tcm.phy.cam.ac.uk. Foundations of Physics, 1991. Web. 16 May 2013.

For the discussion of Dean Radin see "Supernormal." deanradin.com. n.d. Web. 11 October 2014.

On coral castle and ancient monoliths see "The Monoliths", Ancient Aliens, Season 5 Episode 12, history.com.

On Ed Leedskalnin and Coral Castle see Miss Cellania. "Edward Leedskalnin and his Coral Castle." mentalflooss.com. n.d. Web. 11 October 2014. Also see coralcastle.com. Also see Radford, Benjamin; *Mystery of the Coral Castle Explained; Live Science.* November 8, 2013. Livescience.com.

On Robert Cialdini, see Cialdini, Robert; *Pre-Suasion*: A Revolutionary Way to Influence and Persuade; Simon & Schuster; New York, NY; 2016; pg 19. Audio.

For the discussion of magnetoreception in insects, animals, and humans see Bryner, Jeanna. "Humans May Have 'Magnetic' Sixth Sense." livescience.com. livescience, 21 June 2011. Castelvecchi, Davide. "The Compass Within". Scientific American. Jan 2012, Vol. 306 Issue 1, p. 48-53. Baker, Robin R., Janice G. Mather and John H. Kennaugh, Department of Zoology, University of Manchester. *Nature.* Vol 301 Issue 5895. pp. 78-80.

On Stephen Hawking discussing the Butterfly Effect see Hawking, Stephen. *The Universe In A Nutshell.* New York: Bantam Books 2001. 104. Print.

For the quote by Professor Hubbard of Stanford University regarding parallel universes see Hubbard, Scott G. "Space: Definitely Not the Final Frontier." *The Wall Street Journal:* R22, 8 July 2014. Print.

For the image of sun setting on mars see "Sunset on Mars". Image of the day gallery, nasa.gov. Web. 15 January 2015. Credit: NASA/JPL/Texas A&M/Cornell.

Made in the USA
Columbia, SC
29 April 2020